HCG 2.0

Don't Starve · Eat Smart · And Lose

A Modern Adaptation
Of the Traditional HCG Diet

By: Dr. Zach LaBoube

For more information visit...

www.InsideOutWellness.net

Prologue

Medicine is called a practice for a reason. As new technology and research becomes available, treatment protocols evolve, hopefully for the better. Shouldn't the HCG diet be the same? First published in 1954, the traditional HCG diet, as seen on many of your favorite daytime talk shows, including Dr. Oz, has helped millions achieve weight loss success. However, the strict tone and rigid calorie restrictions have been very polarizing. While the concepts and theory that inspired the traditional diet are still very relevant, the protocol itself is still stuck in the 50s and in dire need of revision.

Introducing HCG 2.0, authored and developed by Dr. Zach LaBoube, founder of InsideOut Wellness and Weight Loss, HCG 2.0 utilizes current research into a variety of topics such as low-carb, Ketosis dieting, the high-protein diets of Inuit Cultures and innovative new food statistics such as Estimated Glycemic Load, Fullness Factor and Caloric Ratios to add smart calories to the diet, thus making it a safer, more realistic weight loss option for the working adult.

HCG 2.0 uses a BMR (Basal Metabolic Rate) calculation to determine the amount of calories you're allowed to consume. This is a significant variation from the traditional diet that allows each dieter only 500 calories per day, whether male or female, big or small. Additionally, HCG 2.0 uses precise food chemistry, which was primitive at best when the diet was originally developed, to provide a wider selection of protein options, while also increasing portion size of items higher in nutritional value, but void of empty calories that only contribute to weight gain.

Whether you're looking to lose weight or simply eat better, HCG 2.0 will accommodate. Understand Ketosis and the benefits to low-carb living. Learn the difference between positive and negative calories. Understand how to cut your caloric intake by 200-300 calories per day by simply addressing unnoticed habits, and much more.

There's a smarter way to lose.

Table of Contents

Disclaimer

Please do not interpret anything herein as medical diagnosis or treatment. You should always consult your doctor before beginning a weight loss program.

HCG 2.0

Don't Starve – Eat Smart – And Lose

A modern approach to the traditional HCG diet

When Dr. Simeons developed his protocol for HCG weight loss in 1950's Italy, food was grown fresh, organically. The fish were caught from the sea rather than harvested from breeding pools. The beef was grass fed on the rolling hills of Tuscany. Food is now a business. It's engineered in laboratories with the purpose of extending shelf-life rather than enhancing nutritional content. It's packaged and shipped to all corners of the country like industrial goods. Five-hundred calories today is NOT what it was in 1950's Italy.

When I began working with HCG weight loss, I was a skeptic like many others. A 500 calorie diet didn't seem sustainable and I was reluctant to recommend it to my patients. However, through my own research and witnessing the results of colleagues and mentors already working with HCG, I became a believer. Yet, I was still not fully convinced, primarily due to the restrictions on protein in combination with the inclusion of up to 70 grams of carbohydrates from fruit and bread sticks. This notion of allowing 280 calories from carbs while restricting protein, in an attempt to lose weight, is a direct contradiction to everything we now know of low-carb, Ketosis dieting. Another concern, and an often overlooked component of Dr. Simeons' original HCG protocol, was the fact that his patients were treated on an in-patient basis. Many spent one month to a year at his clinic under constant supervision, removed from the everyday stressors of work, family and activities of daily living that necessitate large amounts of energy and calories. These calorie restrictions cannot realistically be replicated by the average working adult and acts as major deterrent for most would be dieters.

With the decreased nutritional value of our food today, combined with the additional energy requirements of balancing the demands of work, family and life in general, 500 calories just isn't enough. Nor is it reasonable to believe that the calorie requirements be "fixed" for all dieters, as the energy and protein demands of a 6'5" male will be significantly higher than that of a 5'2" woman. As a practitioner, these disconnects were concerning. In the beginning, I was reluctant to deviate from the protocol because I wanted my patients to achieve success. However, as I gained experience with the diet and gathered feedback, I was slowly able to modernize and adapt the 65 year old protocol to accommodate the average working adult.

It's important to remember that the original HCG diet was based entirely on anecdotal results. In fact, 16 years passed between the time Dr. Simeons published his first research article regarding his HCG diet protocol and the time he published his famous manuscript, *Pounds and Inches: a New Approach to Obesity*. During this time he was continuously adding, removing, and revising, while methodically documenting results. The same can be said for medicine in general. It's called a practice for a reason. As new technology and research become available, treatment protocols evolve, hopefully for the better. Likewise, shouldn't the HCG diet be the same? Why wouldn't we use our current research in the biochemistry of Ketosis to question the inclusion of high-sugar, high-carb fruits in Dr. Simeons' original diet? Why wouldn't we use innovative statistics like that of Estimated Glycemic Load, Nutritional Density and Caloric Ratios to increase portion size of food items richer in nutritional value but void of empty calories that only contribute to weight gain? Or, utilize advancements in food technology to incorporate high protein, low-fat, low-carb isolates like whey or soy protein?

These are the questions, amongst many others, that inspired me to deviate from the traditional diet and ultimately create HCG 2.0. Simple food chemistry tells us that 100 grams of chicken has roughly the same caloric value as 200 grams of fish, depending on the variety. If you're not a fish eater, consider bison: a sirloin cut of bison has more protein and half the calories of its beef counterpart. The numbers don't lie. If you're restricting calories to lose weight, would you rather have a small amount of chicken or a filling amount of fish? A *single* beef kabob or *two* bison kabobs? To put it another way, if you had $100, would you rather buy a single shirt from Nordstrom or 2 complete outfits (plus a week's worth of lunch) from Target? It's a matter of smart shopping and budgeting your calories. By adding SMART calories to the diet - high protein, low carb/fat items, and removing the Ketosis inhibiting fruits, I've created a diet that is equally as effective, but safer and more sustainable, thus leading to more widespread success. Bear in mind that I'm not claiming that you'll lose MORE weight on HCG 2.0 than you would on the traditional version, nor was that my goal. My goal was only to provide patients with a smarter, more realistic alternative to the older version. The increase in calories, all from lean protein, provides patients with a more realistic opportunity to succeed resulting in greater optimism and higher completion rates. A diet need not be the undertaking of a lifetime to yield positive results. HCG 2.0 balances a realistic opportunity for success with healthy, rapid weight loss.

Before we begin, it's important to understand that nearly all of the research we have regarding HCG and its role in supporting weight loss is mostly clinical, meaning it is more subjective in nature and not tested in a controlled environment. Additionally, HCG is not a miracle pill that magically makes the unwanted pounds fall off, nor does such pill exist, despite what you might see or hear on TV and radio. HCG requires a restrictive diet. In fact, HCG is not what causes you to lose weight at all. Your weight loss is a result of your decrease in caloric intake and a healthy metabolic process called Ketosis, which is defined and discussed in the pages to follow (page 15 if you'd like to quickly skip ahead). So what then does HCG do and why is it used to accompany this diet?

HCG, as theorized by Dr. Simeons and supported by a substantial collection of clinical research, provides two distinct actions to facilitate your weight loss while on the low calorie phase of the diet and one action following the diet to help you maintain your ideal weight. All three are listed below.

1. HCG **targets your weight loss** so that you maintain muscle mass while strictly losing from abnormal fat deposits.

2. HCG **suppresses appetite** by enhancing Ketosis, which is a process that converts our fat reserves to usable calories allowing us to sustain ourselves on our own stored fat. By summoning calories from stored fat, our body reacts as though it has just consumed a meal thus producing a feeling of satiety and fullness.

3. **Following the low calorie phase** - By acting on a gland in the brain called the hypothalamus, which is responsible for regulating metabolic activity, including hunger and satiety, HCG has the capacity to **"reset" your metabolism allowing you to successfully maintain your weight loss.**

Part 1: The Traditional HCG Diet

Questioning Dr. Simeons

Below are what I found to be the inadequacies of the traditional diet and the areas I believe were in most need of revision. I'm not arguing the effectiveness of the traditional diet, as millions have had tremendous success with it. In fact, I've had many patients tell me that the HCG diet changed their lives. However, I've also had many patients walk out of my office and many drop out of the program because they've found the diet to be too unrealistic. A greater number have said they'd come back at a later date when they had more time and could make it fit into their busy work, family and social schedules. Most don't return. These are the people I'm hoping to help with HCG 2.0. Let's face it, dieting isn't fun, but it should be embraced, not feared. As I said earlier, a weight loss plan need not be the undertaking of a lifetime to yield life-changing results. The revisions I've made to Dr. Simeons original diet, with the assistance and feedback from my patients, will provide the same weight loss results and can be comfortably completed by all.

If you're an HCG purist, and there are many of you out there, then take this with a grain of salt, or whatever allowable spice you'd prefer. Better yet, read with a side of open-mindedness, savoring the ingredients herein to find a tasty combination of the old and the new. Bon appetite! There's a smarter way to lose.

1. **Tone**

   I put this first on the list because I find it to be the biggest roadblock for most would be dieters. What I'm addressing here is the all-or-nothing attitude that is portrayed in Dr. Simeons' manuscript and nearly all of the current literature about the traditional diet. This frightens many patients away and is the typical reason most drop out before completion. Too often, patients on the traditional HCG diet will have consecutive "bad days," and give up. That's foolish and a by-product of this all-or-nothing mentality. My patients will use the word "cheat," but it's not a word I use. There is no "cheating" on any diet, only variations of intensity and success. Any attempt to improve your quality of life should not be feared, nor expected to end in defeat. Don't give up! You can still have success even if you have a couple of "bad days."

2. **Measuring food items in weight rather than in caloric value**

   If you were shopping for a bracelet and your jeweler offered to set your precious stones in 100 grams of gold or 100 grams of copper, you'd be a fool not to choose the gold, right? For the same expense, gold has tremendously more value. The two metals may in fact weigh the same, but they're not remotely equal. The same can be said for the protein options on the traditional diet. You're allowed 100 grams of protein per meal. You may eat an equal portion size of fish one day and beef the next, but the caloric value is quite different. With beef, you're getting roughly the same amount of protein you would in fish (value), but with almost triple the calories (expense). That's not smart shopping. So why not make the two food items "equal?" By equal, I mean equal in calories. Two-hundred grams of white fish is roughly equal to 100 grams of chicken, which, in turn, is equal to about 80 grams of beef. If you're a beef eater, this news may be upsetting, but it's probably time to consider eating more fish. There are plenty of varieties, experiment until you find something you like; and give it some time. Taste is an acquired sense.

3. **The inclusion of high-carb fruit items and bread sticks**

In the traditional HCG diet about 200 of the 500 calories come from fruit and bread sticks, in some situation more. That leaves only 300 calories from lean protein sources. In fact, the numbers on Dr. Simeons' diet don't even add up. Let's look at the scenario below which is an entirely allowable low calorie day on the traditional HCG diet.

Breakfast – Nothing
Lunch - Chicken breast (100g) = 195 calories, tomato = 22, apple = 72, bread stick = 20
       Total = 309 calories and 27.4 grams of carbs
Dinner – Flounder (100g) = 133 calories, onion (1 cup) = 67, orange = 69, bread stick =20
       Total = 289 calories and 37.7 grams of carbs.
          Total for Day = 598 with a substantial 65 grams of carbs

> ➢ Had I substituted a cut of beef for the flounder, the calories would have been over 700.

I bring this up to show you that the traditional diet wasn't as specific as you might think. From the very second I read the original manuscript, the carbs were an immediate concern. If the goal of the diet is to lose weight as quickly as possible, which is the obvious goal of any crash diet, why include carbs? Fruits are great and I would never discourage my patients from eating fruit, but if your objective is to lose weight then they have to be eliminated, as they prevent Ketosis.

Why not apply our current knowledge of zero-carb dieting, and the biochemistry of Ketosis to the traditional diet? Whether Dr. Simeons had any knowledge of Ketosis as a metabolic process when he was practicing is unknown, but he insinuated this Ketogenic effect when he discussed his "steak day." He suggested that if your weight loss begins to stall or if you begin to gain after completing the diet, you should perform a "steak day." This means you eat nothing all day long, starving yourself of all calories, and eat a large steak for dinner. The absence of carbs would likely be enough to reinitiate Ketosis and weight loss.

Sustained Ketosis is the only way to tap into the abnormal fat we tend to store in all the places we don't want it. This is central focus of HCG 2.0.

4. **Limitations on allowable vegetables and serving sizes**

Dr. Simeons' had a very specific list of vegetables that could be consumed on the diet. He claimed that when other vegetables were substituted or when vegetables were mixed, it acted to slow down weight-loss. I have trouble understanding this reasoning, especially considering his vegetable choices. For example, onions are allowed on the traditional diet while bell peppers and broccoli are not. Onions have double the calories and carbs of peppers and nearly triple that of broccoli. Carbs disrupt Ketosis and this is why I believe the weight loss to be inconsistent on the traditional diet. My advice is to do your best to keep your carbs below 30 grams per day and this is best accomplished by selecting green leafy vegetables and limiting root veggies. I hate to limit vegetables at all, but it's necessary to maintain Ketosis. The veggie chart on page 42 is a good resource for comparing your vegetables. They're listed from least carbs to most carbs. The items at the top of the list will be your best options and you're allowed to mix them any way you choose. There is no need to count calories from veggies if you can limit your carb intake to less than 30 grams per day.

5. **Exercise**

Dr. Simeons suggested that exercise was not allowed on his original diet. In fact, as mentioned earlier, many of his patients were treated on an in-patient basis. My advice to patients is to continue doing what you were doing before you started the diet. If you were working out 3 to 5 times prior to starting the diet, continue to do so. If you were doing no exercises prior to starting the diet, try and begin a walking program. Thirty minutes per day is all you need and if you can manage to get this in before breakfast, you'll be surprised at the boost of energy and euphoria it will provide that will last throughout the day. It also will spark your metabolism, thus facilitating greater weight loss.

If you find yourself getting dizzy or lightheaded, obviously take a break. Drink some water and if you feel better you can resume. Additionally, and this will be discussed in more detail later, if your goal is weight loss, vigorous cardio is not the best way to achieve it. Weight loss is best achieved with light-weight/high-repetition weight training, isometric workouts like Yoga, or brisk walking.

6. **Cosmetics and skin care products**

Cosmetics and skin care products have little to no impact on weight loss. You may take slight concern with moisturizers that contain avocado oil or coconut oil, etc., but in the bigger picture, avoiding carbs is what's going to provide you with the most success. It's been my experience that many places that suggest cosmetics are the reason you're not losing weight have sold you some sort of weight loss guarantee. Or maybe they're retailing diet safe lotions or lip balms. As a side note, avoid purchasing your HCG from places that offer guarantees. Medical professionals don't offer guarantees.

7. **Weighing yourself daily**

Dr. Simeons demanded getting on the scale every day. I don't believe this to be productive; in fact, I think it can be harmful. The same reason a financial analyst does not recommend that you look at your stock portfolio on a daily basis, so do I advise my patients not to look at a scale on a daily basis. Your 30-40 day diet is a marathon, not a sprint. If you do the diet properly you'll lose 20+ pounds in 40 days. A single poor day on the scale, in which your weight-loss remains constant or possibly gain, can be demoralizing. This is especially true for women as a result of water retention. Weight loss may stall about the time of ovulation and within a day or two of menstruation. Heat is also a factor in water retention and will affect both men and women. Summers in St. Louis can be scorching and the amount of time you've spent outside in the heat can affect water retention and skew weight loss.

Another reason not to weigh yourself daily is that in the later stages of the diet, weight loss may taper off. However, it's likely that you're actually converting fat mass to lean mass. As muscle tissue weighs more than fat, this may show up as a wash on your bathroom scale, but if you were to analyze body composition, you would see an increase in lean muscle mass and a decrease in fat mass. This is what results in a loss of inches in your problem areas, which you'll notice in the way your clothes are fitting you. This is often overlooked by many dieters and a couple of poor days on the scale can diminish your motivation. Trust in yourself and the program and you'll be thoroughly rewarded. If you still feel it necessary to weigh yourself on a daily basis, then do so, but bear this in mind and allow the scale to tilt a bit either way.

8. New products

Another inadequacy of Dr. Simeons' diet, and by no fault of his own, is that we have an enormous variety of zero-cal/zero-carb products on our store shelves that didn't exist during Dr. Simeons' time. Many practitioners will tell you to avoid these products as they were not included on Dr. Simeons' original diet. My theory on this is do whatever you have to do to keep yourself focused and motivated. If that means having your Diet Coke after lunch, then by all means have at it. After you shed the weight you can address your Diet Coke habit.

The next section will be a recap of Dr. Simeons original manuscript as paraphrased and in his own words. I find the better educated a patient to be on the diet protocol and supporting theories, the greater their success. This is echoed by Dr. Simeons, " In dealing with a disorder in which the patient must take an active part in the treatment, it is, I believe, essential that he or she have an understanding of what is being done and why. Only then can there be intelligent cooperation between physician and patient." (1954)

Dr. Simeons on the Nature of Obesity

I don't intend to re-hash the entire manuscript for you, as it was intended more for other physicians wishing to replicate his protocol rather than patients. However, I do want to share some of his beliefs regarding the nature of obesity and its causes, which unbelievably, are still quite progressive. What I find most compelling is that Dr. Simeons began publishing his research nearly 70 years ago and today we've made little progress in better understanding the nature and cause of obesity. Indeed, it's a very complex issue that has been further exacerbated by the Standard American Diet, appropriately acronymed SAD, but why has there been so little effort towards understanding the biochemistry of obesity and abnormal fat accumulation? There are several conspiracy theories, many outlined in Kevin Trudeau's controversial book, *The Weight-Loss Cure "They" Don't Want You to Know About*; first and foremost being that thin people don't fill hospital beds and therefore don't put money into the pockets of hospitals, insurance providers and pharmaceutical giants. But the fact remains that Dr. Simeons' hypothesis on the nature of obesity is still relatively progressive, as there has been little research to either corroborate or refute.

Dr. Simeons was not only concerned with the cause of obesity and the hope of ultimately "curing" it, but how it was defined by the medical community and society in general.

Prior to reading his manuscript, I was of the belief that if you consume more calories than what you burn off in any given period of time, you gain weight. Weight gain then ultimately leads to obesity. This belief is quite contradictory to Dr. Simeons', who believed over-eating to be a symptom of obesity, rather than its cause. He believed the cause to be a metabolic disorder stemming from a small gland in our brain.

> *"We have grown pretty sure that the tendency to accumulate abnormal fat is a very definite metabolic disorder, much as is, for instance, diabetes. Yet the localization and the nature of this disorder remained a mystery.*
> *Every new approach seemed to lead into a blind alley, and though patients were told that they are fat because they eat too much, we believed that this is neither the whole truth nor the last word in the matter. Refusing to be side-tracked by an all too facile interpretation of obesity, I have always held that overeating is the result of the disorder, not its cause, and that we can make little headway until we can build for ourselves some sort of theoretical structure with which to explain the condition"* (Simeons, Pounds and Inches; A new approach to obesity, 1954).

He would later say in plainer text, "Persons suffering from this particular disorder will get fat regardless of whether they eat excessively, normally or less than normal. A person who is free of the disorder will never get fat, even if he frequently overeats." (1954)

If you're reading this and the above passage rings particularly true, you've probably struggled with weight your entire life. You've likely sat across the dinner table with many a friend and have said to yourself, "I eat no more than anyone else, so why do I gain while they stay the same." This is often echoed in my office among patients. Many don't understand why they continue to gain while co-workers and friends do not. This is where current research has failed in identifying why some people are predisposed to retain more abnormal fat than others. While I'm sympathetic to these patients and find myself more in agreement with Dr. Simeons than disagreement, the point of this book is not to debate the cause of obesity, nor define it as a disease, but merely provide dieters or anyone for that matter, with an aspiration to improve their quality of life with a basic understanding of a diet that works so that they may share in the same success as my patients.

An Interesting Observation

Dr. A.T.W Simeons attended medical school in Germany. His work abroad studying infectious disease, often in impoverished third-world countries, particularly the slums of India, lead him to an interesting observation: that extremely malnourished women were still capable of giving birth to healthy, full weight babies. In further researching this he found **HCG (Human Chorionic Gonadotropin)**, produced by the placenta during pregnancy to be responsible for this phenomenon.

When a woman becomes pregnant, her body is responsible for providing calories to the growing baby for proper development. Just as the baby requires a 24/7 oxygen supply, it also requires a continuous supply of calories. These calories, along with oxygen and other nutrients, are derived from the blood flow that enters the baby's circulation through the umbilical cord. Any interruption in calories, just like any interruption in oxygen would be catastrophic to the development of the baby. Obviously the mother is capable of supplying oxygen in available quantities, but what about calories? The baby can't wait 3-5 hours in between meals for the calories necessary for healthy neonatal development, so the placenta of the mother begins to produce HCG.

HCG is produced in humans only during pregnancy. The sole purpose of the HCG hormone is to provide a continuous calorie source for the growing baby. It does this by acting on a gland in our brain called the hypothalamus. This is discussed more later, but the hypothalamus regulates all metabolic function in the human body and the HCG tells the hypothalamus that additional calories are needed to supply the baby. The hypothalamus then opens up mom's fat reserves, releasing thousands of calories per day into the blood stream, which is then delivered to the baby.

Dr. Simeons theorized that the same concept could be applied to obesity and discovered that when HCG is supplemented, in the absence of a pregnancy, and combined with a low calorie diet, the same effect was produced. The HCG taps into the unwanted fat we tend to store in our bellies, thighs, arms, etc., and converts it into calories in a process called Ketosis. The dieter can then use these calories as an energy source and literally sustain themselves on their own stored fat, resulting in rapid weight loss. Women tend to lose a 1/2 to a full pound per day while men lose up to 2 pounds per day.

It's unclear how much was known about Ketosis when Dr. Simeons' was practicing. There is no mention of it in his manuscript.

Ketosis is a state that exists when your body is deprived of carbohydrates and must resort to its fat stores for energy. Of the foods we eat, carbs are most easily converted into energy. Complex carbohydrates, mostly starches, are broken down to simpler carbohydrates, ultimately glucose, and then converted to ATP (adenosine tri-phosphate) in the citric acid cycle. ATP is the energy exchange used in every cellular process in the human body. It's kind of like the gasoline we put in our cars. Gasoline is refined from more complex hydrocarbons as glucose is from more complex carbohydrates. If we eat excessive calories from carbs, our body stores them away in our fat cells. If we deprive ourselves of carbs, we tap into our fat stores for energy. Think of our fat stores as a bank account. If we're depositing more money than we're spending, or eating more calories than we're burning off, our bank account gets bigger... like our bellies. If we spend more than we deposit, as in the state of low carb dieting and Ketosis, our bank account gets smaller... resulting in weight loss.

A Ketone is an energy source derived from fat and Ketosis is the physiological state in which this takes place. So why is Ketosis such a trendy word in dieting? The first and probably most popular Ketosis Diet was the Atkins diet. In summary, Atkins only stipulation was that you were to consume a minimal amount of carbs. There were relatively few restrictions on fat and protein consumption and it was generally very effective in promoting weight loss. It gained popularity in the mid 90s, but has since lost steam because of its in-sustainability, due the fact that it didn't distinguish between healthy Omega 3 fats and Omega 6 fats. Other Ketosis Diets you may have heard of, or even tried, are the South Beach Diet, Dukan Diet, Paleo Diet, 5/1 protein shake diet and many others. All of these diets are variations of a low carb diet. When you eliminate carbs, your body must tap into fat stores for energy, thus resulting in Ketosis and weight loss.

Carbohydrates are a questionable part of the omnivorous diet of humans, especially highly processed carbs, which have no place whatsoever. There is an abundant amount of research on Inuit cultures and other indigenous tribes throughout the world that eat little to no carbs. These cultures, specifically Inuit, have a high-protein, high-fat diet and during long stretches of time throughout the year go completely without carbs. They experience no teeth decay or heart disease, diabetes is nearly non-existent and there is ZERO obesity. According to Dr. Eric Dewailly, MD, Ph.D, researcher, and Professor of Social and Preventative Medicine at Laval University, "The traditional Inuit diet is fats and proteins, no sugar at all. It is probably one of the healthiest diets you can have. The human body is built for that. "(2007).

If this high-protein, high-fat diet is so healthy, why don't we hear more about its positive effects? Probably for a lot of reasons, some relating to our "for-profit" health care system, others relating to the simple fact that the word "fat" carries such a negative connotation that doctors are reluctant to recommend it. But don't be fooled, a high-protein, high-fat diet, balanced with a 1:1 ratio of Omega 3s to Omega 6s is what we're built for, as Dr. Dewailly says.

The traditional HCG diet, as practiced by Dr. Simeons, is a "mildly" Ketogenic Diet with the addition of the HCG hormone. The traditional diet consists of adequate protein, low fats and adequate carbs combined with the HCG hormone supplement. There is a slight discrepancy in the research regarding the amount of carbs one can consume and still maintain Ketosis. Keep in mind that Ketosis isn't all-or-nothing. There are depths and stages; less carbs equals greater Ketosis which in turn results in more rapid weight loss. Some research suggests that Ketosis can be achieved at .5 grams of carbs per pound. So for example, if you weigh 180 pounds, you can consume 90 grams of carbs and achieve Ketosis. Others research says you must consume less than 50 grams per day to achieve Ketosis. The Atkins diet, as we discussed earlier, allows for only 20 grams of carbs. The traditional HCG diet allowed between 60 and 80, which, by any standard, is at the high end of Ketosis. Limiting carbs is the absolute most important thing you can do to accelerate/maintain your weight loss. And, if you're like most, this will be the most difficult part. Not simply because we crave carbs, but because starches are such a staple in our diet that we almost cannot imagine a meal without them.

Starches, which are complex carbohydrates in comparison to sugars, which are simple carbohydrates, make for cheap filler. I grew up in a family of five and while we were very middle class, we lived on a pretty strict budget. This probably won't be much of a surprise to many readers as you will relate, but my mother could make a single pound of hamburger last two meals. She did so with starches; potatoes, noodles, bread, etc. This is how many of us were raised and this habitual component of our diet, or how we ate as children, is a powerful motivator as to how we eat as adults. The starch habit is a perfect example of this. The problem with starches, and more so with simple carbohydrates like those in fruit, is that they are so rapidly digested that the rush of incoming fuel cannot be fully metabolized and these calories ultimately end up stored as fat. This is ok as children because we're more active, but if we continue to consume the same percentage of carbs as adults we'll gain weight because our activity level and metabolic rate decrease significantly.

Additionally, Ketosis has a significant effect on the amount of hunger you'll experience on the diet. When your body is comfortably in a state of Ketosis, as it is when limiting carbs to 30 grams per day, you'll be supplied with ample amounts of ketone calories from stored fat; this will not only provide you with sufficient energy, but will mediate hunger. When you're fluctuating in and out of Ketosis, as you often will on the traditional diet, you won't be consistently supplied with ketone calories and you'll experience both lethargy and intermittent hunger.

By eliminating the high-sugar fruits and bread sticks that were allowed on the traditional diet, and replacing those calories with lean protein, you've already brought your carb intake to below 30 grams per day, which will comfortably maintain Ketosis by any research standard. This is the key to HCG 2.0. The HCG then expedites and targets Ketosis by "unlocking" our abnormal fat stores. It's important to note that the **HCG is NOT what causes your weight loss**. The weight loss is derived from your low calorie, Ketosis diet. Then why add HCG? Look at it this way, if Ketosis is the door that houses our abnormal fat, HCG is the "key." Before I elaborate, we need to discuss fat, its role in the human body, both good and bad, and why it accumulates in some of us more than others.

Three Types of Fat

The word fat immediately strikes up a negative connotation, and deservedly so; am I right? Nobody wants to be called fat and in the 80s, fat was declared our enemy. There was a low-fat version of everything on our store shelves from butter to salad dressing, even eggs. Many of these products are still on our shelves today, but I would take caution. Typically, the fat is replaced with processed sugars to maintain flavor. Given current research, the processed sugars should be considerably more feared than fat.

As a side note, you'll find these trends to be a recurring theme in the food industry and more a result of capitalism rather than nutritional research. Michael Pollan does a great job of exposing this in his book, *In Defense of Food; an Eaters Manifesto*. Pollan, a journalist whom I have tremendous respect, is an unbiased observer of the food industry. Often, his research exposes the food industry for what it is… a business; therefore more concerned with profits rather than the health and wellbeing of its consumers. If you're curious, the hot trend now is Gluten free. There are entire aisles in the super market dedicated to Gluten free products. If you're one of the few that suffer from Celiac Disease, which is a condition that causes an adverse inflammatory reaction to Gluten, your dinner options have never been better, but for the rest of us it's just another fad; an area of revenue opportunity and potential growth for the giants of the food manufacturing industry.

I digress. Let's get back to the discussion of fat and its three variations within the human body. What may surprise you is that most fat is necessary… and good.

There are three types of fats, **visceral** or **structural fats, normal fats** and **abnormal fats**. The **visceral,** also known as **structural fats** are the soft elastic fats that surround our internal organs, providing them cushioning and protection. These essential fats also protect your bones and arteries and keep your skin healthy and taut.

The second type of fat is what is known as **normal fat** reserves. These fats are called upon freely when nutritional intake becomes insufficient. These fats are stored all over the body. Fats, as compared to protein or carbohydrates, pack the highest caloric value into the smallest amount of space so fuel is economically stored for all of your body's needs. These normal fats are healthy fat reserves. Even if your body stores these to capacity, it does not result in obesity.

Abnormal fat is the enemy. Abnormal fat wears the mask and rides a black horse and whom we would like to avoid at all costs. It's unclear why these abnormal fat reserves accumulate in the body with absolutely no uniformity from one individual to the next. It's hypothesized that these fats act as some sort of primitive survival mechanism that protect us from long periods of diminished food supplies such as long winters or famine, conditions that in the United States, we don't often see. There is also research suggesting that these abnormal fat cells develop as children. Some children develop more while others develop less, maybe as a result of poor childhood nutrition. While the number of these fat cells remains constant as we get older, the size of the abnormal fat cells can grow and grow and grow. The research is unclear, but it's logical to assume that it is of high importance to start your children off with good eating habits in order to limit the amount of abnormal fat cells. If you're obese as a child and/or adolescent, maintaining a healthy weight as an adult will always be a struggle.

Of these three types of fats, abnormal fats are the most difficult to target through traditional dieting. According to Dr. Simeons, "When an obese patient tries to reduce by starving himself, he will first lose his normal fat reserves. When these are exhausted he begins to burn up structural fat, and only as a last resort will the body yield its abnormal reserves, though by that time the patient usually feels so weak and hungry that the diet is abandoned. It is just for this reason that obese patients complain that when they diet they lose the wrong fat. They feel famished and tired and their face becomes drawn and haggard, but their belly, hips, thighs and upper arms show little improvement. The fat they have come to detest stays on and the fat they need to cover their bones gets less and less. Their skin wrinkles and they look old and miserable. And that is one of the most frustrating and depressing experiences a human being can have." (1954). If you're reading at home and you've tried several diets with little or no success, this will ring true.

These abnormal fat cells were the focus of Dr. Simeons' research. He believed that the calories stored within were what allowed the malnourished women he observed in India to give birth to healthy, full-weight babies. But the question remained, why were these calories only accessible by pregnant women? Upon further research, he found HCG to be the "key."

The Hypothalamus and Its Role

Dr. Simeons theorized that HCG acted on a gland in the brain called the hypothalamus. The hypothalamus is an extremely small gland located deep within the brain. It weighs only about 4 grams and makes up less than 1% of the total mass of our brains. However, it provides several vital functions including the regulation of sleep, thirst, temperature, **hunger and satiety**, reproduction, and some more primitive aspects of behavior. In fact, most functions of the hypothalamus are of a very primitive nature. The hypothalamus also controls our thyroid gland which regulates our metabolism, establishing our BMR or Basal Metabolic Rate. Your BMR is the amount of calories you need to maintain normal "at rest" body function.

Unfortunately, most of the research on hypothalamic function has not been performed on humans, but on animals, as the gland is located deep within the human brain and lesions in this area are very rare. In animals, primarily laboratory rats, a lesion is induced on various parts of the hypothalamus and behavior is observed and tests are performed. Some of this research existed when Dr. Simeons was articulating his hypothesis, but much was not. The passage you're about to read regarding hypothalamic function and obesity was taken from the Neuroanatomy Course Book from the University of Wisconsin. Set Point Theory of Obesity, which we'll soon define, was in its infancy when Dr. Simeons was developing his theories and there is no known research establishing a connection to Dr. Simeons and Set Point Theory of weight management.

The largest and most prominent of the nuclei in the medial part of the tuberal region is the ventromedial nucleus. One important function that has been attributed to the ventromedial nucleus is control of eating. Bilateral lesions of the ventromedial nucleus in animals and probably humans as well, result in overeating (hyperphagia) and extreme obesity (Fig. 4) as well as a chronically irritable mood and increase in aggressive behavior (termed hypothalamic rage). By contrast, bilateral lesions in the lateral hypothalamic area result in anorexia (lack of appetite). Animals with lesions in this area may die of starvation. As a result of these lesion studies (along with supporting stimulation studies), the ventromedial nucleus has been referred to as a satiety center and the lateral hypothalamic area as a feeding center. It has been postulated that these opposing centers define a "set point" for body weight: the set point theory of weight control. According to this theory, when body weight goes below the set point, the lateral hypothalamus is activated and appetite is increased; when body weight goes above the set point, the ventromedial nucleus is activated and appetite is decreased. This theory was questioned in the past, but recent evidence has been obtained that supports an integrative role of the ventromedial nucleus and lateral hypothalamic area in body weight control: their neurons respond to glucose, free fatty acid and insulin levels in a manner consistent with the set point theory, and activity levels in the two nuclei display a strict reciprocal relationship that is appropriately correlated with the level of hunger or satiety." (University of Wisconsin (n.d.). *Hypothalamus)*

As you can see from the literature above, there is agreement in the medical community that the hypothalamus is, in fact, regarded as playing a critical role in obesity. Dr. Simeons believed a poorly functioning hypothalamus to be the reason some people retain more abnormal fat than others. Again, there is no known connection to Dr. Simeons and Set Point Theory and there is no mention of it in his manuscript, but I believe a correlation can be made between Set Point Theory and Dr. Simeons belief that HCG can effectively "re-set" one's metabolism to alter ones set point for the better.

Set point theory states that each and every one of us has our own "ideal" weight. This is the weight that our body is comfortable with and strives to maintain despite the number of calories we consume and regardless of our energy expenditures. Given this theory, any attempts to lose weight, thus falling below our ideal weight or "set point" will be met with resistance. This resistance is a survival mechanism that leaps into action every time we experience a decrease in caloric intake. You may have also heard this referred to as "starvation mode" which will be mentioned again later. This seems reasonable, doesn't it? In fact, if you're a yo-yo dieter like so many of us, you may have experienced this for yourself. Gain, lose. Gain, lose. Like a yo-yo.

The other side of the coin regarding Set Point Theory, and the reason it hasn't been accepted by many in the medical profession, including myself to a certain degree, is that it doesn't have an off button. For example, when an individual becomes dangerously obese, their satiety response doesn't kick in and slow down their eating habits. In fact, the opposite happens. The morbidly obese continue to gain and gain.

I may have veered off track here as I committed to you earlier that I would not debate the cause of obesity as it is too complex and not really worth our time, but I'd like to share my opinion on Set Point Theory, which both supports and challenges the concept and may shed some light on why we are predisposed to retain fat... some of us more than others.

Human physiology, all the normal metabolic processes going on underneath our skin, happens with the single objective of maintaining our long-term survival. In fact, I shouldn't limit this to just human physiology but life in general, from the smallest creatures to the largest creatures, plant or animal. We've evolved because of our ability to adapt to our environment. As humans, the past million years, give or take a few, have been spent hunting and foraging to provide our bodies and brains with enough calories to propagate the survival of our species. This means we've become very efficient with the utilization and expenditure of the calories we consume, particularly protein. Only in the last two to three thousand years have we been able to manipulate our environments to provide us with an excess of calories, examples being agriculture and refined grains for producing bread. However, our physiology remains a million years behind, still in survival mode, stock piling calories away in fat to survive the winter. This means that until our primitive human physiology develops an innate capability of regulating our calorie consumption in correspondence with an OVER-abundant food supply, our conscience brains and our will power will have to do it for us... the gland likely to take responsibility for this is the hypothalamus.

The hypothalamus could do this in one of two ways: by either regulating our satiety response or by limiting the amount of calories we deposit into our abnormal fat reserves. Dr. Simeons believed a combination of both to be correct as the obese patient, with a higher tendency to retain abnormal fat, will produce a skewed satiety response, resulting in over-eating. This could certainly be argued, along with the proverbial chicken or the egg (both of which are acceptable food items on the HCG 2.0 Diet), but we'll save that argument for a later date. Let's get to the point and FINALLY address HCG and its role in weight loss and effectively maintaining it.

When we diet or decrease our caloric intake to levels lower than what we are accustomed to and lower than what we are burning off, our hypothalamus typically targets normal fats, structural fats, and lean muscle to supplement this decrease in calories. That's right, you heard me correct. Our body will steal calories from lean muscle before it will tap into our abnormal fat reserves in an attempt to re-establish its "set point." There have been several studies, dating back to 2003, the earlier days of gastric bypass surgery that illustrate this effect. In 2012 a study conducted by Department of Internal Medicine, Division of Cardiology, William Beaumont Hospital, concluded that, "After bariatric surgery, those patients losing weight at the greatest rate appear to have accelerated losses of both lean and fat mass. Few patients maintain lean body mass after bariatric surgery, despite self-reported participation in conventional exercise programs. These data suggest the need for more aggressive interventions to preserve lean body mass during the weight loss phase after Roux-en-Y gastric bypass surgery." (Zaleson, Franklin, Lillystone, Shamon, Krause, Chengelis, Mucci & Shaheen, 2010)

In 2010 a similar study by The Center for Research on Micronutrients, Universidade Federal do Rio de Janeiro concluded the same, "Bariatric surgery proved to be effective in reducing total body mass and body fat at every time interval. However, dietary measures emphasizing adequate protein intake may be implemented in order to reduce loss of LBM (Lean Body Mass) and, coupled with frequent physical activity, may help curtail the impact the surgery has on morphological variables." (de Aquino, Pereira, de Souza, Sobrinho & Ramalho, 2012) This reinforces the fact that decreasing calories as we do during traditional dieting leads to a decrease in muscle mass, which is not the goal of any dieter. This certainly does not help from an aesthetic standpoint and it's unhealthy.

Any reduction in lean muscle tissue as a result of dieting is entirely counter-productive and should be avoided at all costs. The average dieter is concerned with the accumulation of fat in problem areas such as bellies, thighs, arms, etc., and this is always the most difficult weight to lose. If you've attempted multiple diets in the past with little or no success, you're probably nodding your head in agreement at this very moment.

This is the role of HCG: to target your weight loss so that you maintain muscle mass while strictly losing from abnormal fat that is stored in problem areas, i.e. bellies, arms, thighs, neck,. Fat, as we've already established, is the body's most efficient way to store energy. One gram of fat contains 9 calories as opposed to carbohydrates which contain 4 calories per gram and protein, which also contain just 4 calories per gram. A secondary effect of HCG, as observed by Dr. Simeons, is that by "unlocking" these abnormal fat reserves, thus kick starting Ketosis, an additional 1500-4000 calories per day of stored fat is entering the blood stream and available to you as a source of useable energy. This allows you to; quite literally, sustain yourself on your own stored fat, thus inducing rapid weight loss. Additionally, these calories derived from Ketosis act on our satiety response just as calories that we've eaten from a meal, which produces a feeling of satisfaction, satiety and/or fullness. In fact, many pregnant women will tell you that during specific times in their pregnancy, typically early in the second trimester, their appetite is diminished and they feel full faster (see graph indicating HCG concentrations during pregnancy). This is likely an effect of the HCG and a similar effect is experienced by HCG dieters beginning at approximately the middle of the second week and lasting for 10 to 15 days throughout the middle of the diet. These effects begin to diminish towards the end of the diet as you begin acclimate to the hormone, rendering it less effective, which is the reason Dr. Simeons kept his patients on a 30-40 day cycle of the diet. Rather than increase dosages of HCG, the dieter is removed from the diet for roughly the same amount of time they were on it and after following the semi-restrictive maintenance diet, they can resume again.

weeks since LMP	mIU/mL
3	5 – 50
4	5 – 426
5	18 – 7,340
6	1,080 – 56,500
7 – 8	7,650 – 229,000
9 – 12	25,700 – 288,000
13 – 16	13,300 – 254,000
17 – 24	4,060 – 165,400
25 – 40	3,640 – 117,000
Non-pregnant females	<5.0
Postmenopausal females	<9.5

As a side note, in relation to the graph above taken from Wikipedia showing HCG concentration throughout pregnancy, after giving birth, women have a short window in which to lose their baby weight. Have you ever said to a friend or family member following her pregnancy, "I can't believe how quickly you got your shape back?" Maybe you've even experienced this for yourself? It's likely a by-product of the remaining HCG in your system. If the weight is not lost quickly following pregnancy, it will be an uphill battle. Certainly there are contributing factors such as age and breast-feeding, but the HCG shouldn't be discounted. Additionally, and in relation to pregnancy, the skin rebounds very quickly. Pregnant women may show the appearance of stretch marks, but they don't have an excess of loose, flabby skin following birth. Many HCG dieters who have lost a considerable amount of weight experience the same, positive effect.

I'll also add that many HCG dieters experience a certain amount of euphoria while on the diet. It's certainly possible that this is a result of getting healthy, but the HCG could be a factor as well. "It is no exaggeration to say that the flooding of the female body with HCG is by far the most spectacular hormonal event in pregnancy. It has an enormous protective importance for mother and child." (1954)

To summarize, let's review the overall effects of HCG in facilitating weight loss during the low calorie phase of your diet.

What does the HCG do to help me lose weight?

1. **Targets weight loss**, allowing you to lose fat and inches from problem areas while maintaining lean muscle mass. People tend to overlook the "inches" part. It's a very under-appreciated benefit to HCG. In the later stages of the diet, weight loss will diminish, but you'll actually see a conversion of fat mass to lean mass. Muscle weighs more than fat, which disguises your actual weight loss. I had one patient that was disappointed that she only lost 19 pounds, but after measuring, she lost a total of 39 inches... that's over three feet!!!

2. **Facilitates and prolongs ketosis** by tapping into abnormal fat reserves, allowing you to sustain yourself on your own stored fat.

3. **Suppresses appetite** by introducing Ketone calories, or calories derived from our stored fat, into our system. This results in an insulin response as though we've just eaten a meal. A secondary effect of insulin is it tells our brains we're satiated.

The effects listed above are the primary contributors to your weight loss, or better said, fat loss. The other claim made by Dr. Simeons, and what many find most controversial, including myself, is that HCG "resets" your metabolism allowing you to comfortably maintain your weight loss. This is probably the most polarizing aspect of the diet for several reasons. The first and most obvious being that maintaining a healthy weight is predominantly, some would say entirely, dependant on the decisions you make following the diet. I like to tell patients that everyone will lose weight on the low calorie phase of the diet, but whether you keep the weight off is entirely up to you. Perhaps this is better said by Dr. Yoni Freedoff, blogger of www.weightymatters.ca, "The more weight you'd like to permanently lose, the more of your lifestyle you'll need to permanently change." (2007) This doesn't mean I've completely discredited Dr. Simeons' theory that HCG "resets" your metabolism, but I feel there are many contributing factors to maintaining a healthy weight following your HCG diet as we'll discuss.

Whether you've done the diet before or if you're reading about HCG for the first time, it's necessary to have an understanding of the original HCG Diet developed by Dr. Simeons. Keep in mind that Dr. Simeons' patients were treated on an in-patient basis. I've mentioned this before and I bring this up again for two reasons, the first being that patients being treated on an in-patient basis are removed from the stress and anxiety of daily life. Not only does this significantly impact calorie expenditures, but it also detracts from the amount of focus you can give to the diet. Think about it, do any of us have 30 to 40 days to dedicate to a diet? Unlikely! If you're the norm, you're juggling work, family, kids, husband, wife, and you're lucky to find a second for yourself. I tell patients on a daily basis that the unhealthy foods we eat are not our foods of choice but our foods of convenience.   I remind you of this so that you can understand why I was continuously revising the diet, adding lean protein, adding more lean protein while reducing carbs, and finally giving busy people an opportunity to succeed.

The Basics of the Traditional HCG Diet

The following is a combination of Dr. Simeons' original text and my paraphrasing of his text. My paraphrasing is written in plain text, and language from Dr. Simeons' original manuscript is *italicized*.

Phase 1 or P1 of HCG Diet:
Overeating (Loading) Phase: Days 1 and 2

This phase consists of the first two days of the traditional HCG diet developed by Dr. Simeons. You'd begin taking HCG as directed. These days would be spent overeating on as much fatty food as you could consume with no restrictions. This seems counter-productive, but we'll discuss the relevance of this later, when I introduce HCG 2.0.

One cannot keep a patient comfortably on 500 Calories unless his normal fat reserves are reasonably well stocked. It is for this reason that every case, even those that are actually gaining must eat to capacity of the most fattening food they can get down.

Phase 2 or P2 of HCG Diet:
Very Low Calorie Diet (VLCD) Phase: 23 to 40 days

After completion of the loading days, you would begin the Very Low Calorie Diet (VLCD). Again, keep in mind that most of Dr. Simeons' patients were treated on an in-patient basis and under continuous observation. You don't need such extreme calorie restrictions to achieve success. Just be smart with your calories.

The VLCD, as detailed in Dr. Simeon's original manuscript is listed below. There was no variation to this protocol in terms of calories and allowable foods whatsoever. The diet was 100% consistent regardless of age, gender, height and weight. What's listed below is copied directly from Dr. Simeons' manuscript, *Pounds and Inches; A New Approach to Obesity* (1954).

Breakfast: Tea or coffee in any quantity without sugar. Only one tablespoonful of milk allowed in 24 hours. Saccharin or Stevia may be used.

Lunch:

1. *100 grams of veal, beef, chicken breast, fresh white fish, lobster, crab, or shrimp. All visible fat must be carefully removed before cooking, and the meat must be weighed raw. It must be boiled or grilled without additional fat. Salmon, eel, tuna, herring, dried or pickled fish are not allowed. The chicken breast must be removed from the bird.*
2. *One type of vegetable only to be chosen from the following: spinach, chard, chicory, beet-greens, green salad, tomatoes, celery, fennel, onions, red radishes, cucumbers, asparagus, cabbage.*
3. *One breadstick (grissini) or one Melba toast.*
4. *An apple or a handful of strawberries or one-half grapefruit or orange.*

Dinner: The same four choices as lunch.

The fruit or the breadstick may be eaten between meals instead of with lunch or dinner, but not more than four items listed for lunch and dinner may be eaten at one meal.

No medicines or cosmetics other than lipstick, eyebrow pencil and powder may he used without special permission

Every item in the list is gone over carefully, continually stressing the point that no variations other than those listed may be introduced. All things not listed are forbidden, and the patient is assured that nothing permissible has been left out. The 100 grams of meat must he scrupulously weighed raw after all visible fat has been removed. To do this accurately the patient must have a letter-scale, as kitchen scales are not sufficiently accurate and the butcher should certainly not be relied upon. Those not uncommon patients, who feel that even so little food is too much for them, can omit anything they wish. 22

There is no objection to breaking up the two meals. For instance having a breadstick and an apple for breakfast or before going to bed, provided they are deducted from the regular meals. The whole daily ration of two breadsticks or two fruits may not be eaten at the same time, nor can any item saved from the previous day be added on the following day. In the beginning patients are advised to check every meal against their diet sheet before starting to eat and not to rely on their memory. It is also worth pointing out that any attempt to observe this diet without HCG will lead to trouble in two to three days. We have had cases in which patients have proudly flaunted their dieting powers in front of their friends without mentioning the fact that they are also receiving treatment with HCG. They let their friends try the same diet, and when this proves to be a failure - as it necessarily must - the patient starts raking in unmerited kudos for superhuman willpower.

It should also be mentioned that two small apples weighing as much as one large one never the less have a higher caloric value and are therefore not allowed though there is no restriction on the size of one apple. Some people do not realize that chicken breast does not mean the breast of any other fowl, nor does it mean a wing or drumstick. The most tiresome patients are those who start counting calories and then come up with all manner of ingenious variations which they compile from their little books. When one has spent years of weary research trying to make a diet as attractive as possible without jeopardizing the loss of weight, culinary geniuses who are out to improve their unhappy lot are hard to take.

Concluding a Course

When the three days of dieting after the last injection are over, the patients are told that they may now eat anything they please, except sugar and starch provided they faithfully observe one simple rule. This rule is that they must have their own portable bathroom-scale always at hand, particularly while traveling. They must without fail weight themselves every morning as they get out of bed, having first emptied their bladder. If they are in the habit of having breakfast in bed, they must weigh before breakfast.

It takes about 3 weeks before the weight reached at the end of the treatment becomes stable, i.e. does not show violent fluctuations after an occasional excess. During this period patients must realize that the so-called carbohydrates, that is sugar, rice, bread, potatoes, pastries etc, are by far the most dangerous. If no carbohydrates whatsoever are eaten, fats can be indulged in somewhat more liberally and even small quantities of alcohol, such as a glass of wine with meals, does no harm, but as soon as fats and starch are combined things are very liable to get out of hand. This has to be observed very carefully during the first 3 weeks after the treatment is ended otherwise disappointments are almost sure to occur.

What you see italicized above is the original HCG diet as published by Dr. Simeon in his manuscript *Pounds and Inches; A new approach to obesity.* To say the least, it's very restrictive. So restrictive in fact that adhering to it 100% is almost unrealistic to the point of being counter-productive. This is what I was referring to earlier when we discussed the tone of his manuscript. At first glance, many will lose interest because it sounds just too unreasonable. I've had this conversation with many patients who have found me through Google search and made appointments. After a consultation on the diet, I frequently found myself educating patients more on food items and beverages that they could "cheat" with and still get positive results, rather than the food items listed on the original diet. This is what inspired me to question the original diet and ultimately put pen to paper and write this adaptation. Adding smart calories to the diet, which you'll see below, provides **greater optimism/enthusiasm, more satiety and greater sustainability.**

HCG 2.0

I've done little to change this phase of the traditional HCG diet other than put more emphasis on fats rather than carbs. The loading phase is necessary to enhance abnormal fat breakdown, but it also provides incentive to begin the diet. Many will schedule their two loading days to coincide with Holidays or vacations. Super Bowl Sunday and Thanksgiving are the two favorites I see in my practice. One would generally never consider beginning a diet on Thanksgiving, but what better time to overload on fatty foods than Thanksgiving Day and Black Friday. And why not; eat with a purpose!

Eat as much fatty food as you want during these two days. In fact, overload yourself on fats. Still be cautious of sugar and carbs. These are not forbidden in the loading phase of your diet, but the focus should be on fats. Try and get a good mix of Omega 3 fats (healthy fats such as avocado, fish and nuts) and Omega 6 fats which are your animal fats and dairy. Enjoy yourself; this is your last hoorah! This isn't to say that you'll never again eat any of your favorites, but you'll eat them intelligently, balanced with a healthy whole food diet.

Beginning - The first two days that you begin taking your HCG supplement, it's necessary to overload on fatty foods. This may seem counter-productive, but it serves three purposes. First, the sudden fat overload causes your hypothalamus to spring into action by alerting the body to begin attacking fats, essentially jump starting the diet. Secondly, the excess fat provides an immediate calorie reserve to mediate your hunger during the early stages of the diet, allowing the HCG ample time to tap into your fat stores, which can take up to 5-7 days. Finally, as we discussed earlier regarding Set Point Theory, keep in mind that human physiology exists for our long term survival and any sudden decrease in calories can alarm the body into "starvation mode." During starvation mode, your body actually becomes more efficient with its calories and more determined to store away fat, assuming that there is a scarcity in food supply. This is why dieting is so difficult. Not only are we battling our own poor eating habits, but a physiological pre-disposition to retain fat. Loading on fats for two days causes your liver enzymes to spike which is theorized to prevent the body from entering this starvation mode. By the time your liver enzymes return to normal levels, the HCG has already tapped into your fat reserves and is providing you with supplemental calories thus bypassing starvation mode, which facilitates more rapid weight loss.

It's quite possible to gain 2 to 3 pounds during the loading phase. Don't let that discourage you. It will be lost quickly. **To Summarize...**

1. The sudden fat overload causes your hypothalamus to spring into fat burning mode, essentially jump starting the diet.
2. The excess fat provides an immediate calorie reserve to mediate your hunger during the early stages of the diet, allowing the HCG to tap into your fat stores, which can take up to 5-7 days. .
3. Overloading on fats fools the body into bypassing starvation mode thus accelerating weight loss.

> ➤ *If you can keep the emphasis on fats, you've got the green light to get after it. A sweet desert certainly won't hurt you, but focus on fats. Get your dairy and cheese fix in because you won't get any on the low calorie phase.*

> ➤ *If you've had a cholecystectomy, or other gall bladder issues, DO NOT attempt the loading days without first consulting your physician. I've worked with patients in the past with these issues and we've typically extended the two heavy loading days to 3 to 4 moderate loading days and most have had little complications and success, but don't attempt this on your own.*

Suggestions for loading

BREAKFAST: *eggs and sausage or bacon*, toast with **peanut butter**, *real butter* and or *cream cheese*

LUNCH: *cheeseburger with mayonnaise*, **avocado slices** and *chili-cheese fries*

DINNER: **baked salmon**, *loaded baked potato with cheese and sour cream*, veggies of your choice with *melted cheese*

SNACKS: **nuts**, chips with **guacamole**, celery with **peanut butter**, canned **tuna w/avocado slices**

> ➤ **Healthy Omega 3 fats are bolded above.** *Omega 6 fats are italicized.* You need to begin to familiarize yourself with these as they will be critical in maintaining your weight loss and optimal health.

Phase 2: Low Calorie Diet **30-40 Days**

It's recommended by Dr. Simeons that this stage must be done for a minimum of 21 days to achieve the desired effect on the hypothalamus gland allowing you to maintain your new weight. I don't have any evidence to contradict this, nor is there much evidence in support, but I will say that a healthy lifestyle is habitual and the longer you can refrain from the foods that facilitated your weight gain, the better chance you'll have at keeping weight off.

I'll also add that taste is an acquired sense. The more vegetables you eat, the better they'll taste. This is something to keep in mind if you have children. It is so important to expose your children to healthy foods such as fruits, vegetables and Omega 3 fats like avocado early and often as they'll be assured to like them as an adult. I have a great photo of my lovely little niece in her Care Bear Halloween costume eating broccoli off of my plate while holding a giant bag of candy. Sure, she likes her sweets, but even at the age of 13 months, she has already acquired a taste for her veggies.

The low calorie phase of the diet is where the original protocol of the diet and HCG 2.0 begin to diverge. In understanding that the ultimate goal of every diet is to lose weight, and like any American seeking immediate gratification, we want to lose weight as quickly as possible. However, with high risk there is high reward. With this in mind, the risk (your financial investment + your ability to sacrifice/sustain/persevere) and the reward (weight loss) are determined by you. It is necessary to count calories, but only in regard to protein as there are no overt carbs or starches allowed. You will not count calories from vegetables, but you will be conscience of their carb content as you are not to exceed 30 grams of carbs in a given day. Nor will you overtly count calories from fats, as the fat you consume on the low calorie phase is only a by-product of your protein choices. The fruit that was allowed on the original HCG diet has been replaced on HCG 2.0 by protein-- the leaner the better as indicated by the P/CF (PFC) number.

The PFC number is used to rank your protein options from best to adequate. It's a simple statistic that can be calculated by any dieter with a calculator or smart phone and was inspired by some progressive research and statistics from NutrtitionalData.com (ND). There are several good websites full of nutritional information, but a majority of them simply regurgitate food labels and offer little analysis of the foods we eat, and even more seldom do they offer original content or research. Nutritional Data is on the cutting edge in this regard and some of its innovative statistics were a big inspiration to me in writing HCG 2.0.

Bear with me for a quick second as I make a baseball analogy. For my female readers, don't lose interest just yet. You may find this paragraph useful if the subject of baseball surfaces with a date or a gentlemen sitting across from you at an airport bar. Better yet, maybe you're a fan yourself. Needless to say, I'm a baseball fan. When I was a kid, there were just a handful of stats used to compare baseball players and the contributions they made to their respective teams. Position players were judged primarily by batting average, home runs and RBIs. Pitchers had their own set of stats such as ERA and strikeouts, and these were the simple stats that all players were measured. Now, baseball has gone high tech using what's called Sabrmetrics, derived from the acronym SABR, Society of American Baseball Research. I know, even the name sounds complicated. However, these extraordinarily advanced statistics are now the norm for player evaluation and scouting and they've added a tremendous amount of intelligence to the game. NutritionalData.com is the Sabrmetrics of the foods we eat.

They've stepped outside the "cereal box" and created an entirely new and innovative way to evaluate our foods using research from the USDA National Nutrient Database for Standard Reference, Daily Reference Values (DRVs), Reference Daily Intakes (RDIs), published research and recommendations from the FDA. Nutritional Data then compresses all of this research into a variety of new food stats such as Nutritional Density, Estimated Glycemic Load, Inflammation Factor, Caloric Ratio, Fullness Factor and many more. This all sounds very complicated, but in a healthy, Omega-3-friendly "nutshell," what it all boils down to is what we already know from our Inuit friends: carbs are bad and high protein, high fat diets with an equal ratio of Omega 3 fats to Omega 6 fats are good. All the Italicized information below was taken directly from www.NutritionalData.com and gives you a general idea of the information they provide.

ESTIMATED GLYCEMIC LOAD™*Glycemic load is a way of expressing a food or meal's effect on blood-sugar levels. Nutrition Data's patent-pending Estimated Glycemic Load™ (eGL) is available for every food in the database as well as for custom foods, meals, and recipes in your Pantry.*

How to interpret the values: Experts vary on their recommendations for what your total glycemic load should be each day. A typical target for total Estimated Glycemic Load is 100 or less per day. If you have diabetes or metabolic syndrome, you might want to aim a little lower. If you are not overweight and are physically active, a little higher is acceptable.

IF (INFLAMMATION FACTOR) RATING™*The IF (Inflammation Factor) Rating™ estimates the inflammatory or anti-inflammatory potential of individual foods or combinations of* *foods by calculating the net effect of different nutritional factors, such as fatty acids, antioxidants, and glycemic impact.*

How to interpret the values: Foods with positive IF Ratings are considered anti-inflammatory and those with negative IF Ratings are considered inflammatory. The higher the number, the stronger the effect. The goal is to balance negative foods with positive foods so that the combined rating for all foods eaten in a single day is positive.

Prior to researching and exploring Nutritional Data's website, my patients and I were already having success in removing the high carb foods on the traditional HCG diet and substituting them with high protein foods. The validation came when I realized that ALL of the foods we were substituting into the old diet ranked exceptionally well in categories such as Estimated Glycemic Load, Inflammation Factor, Fullness Factor and many more

Estimated Glycemic Load (eGL), for example, is an excellent indicator of a food items ability to maintain Ketosis. The closer an item is to zero, the better, meaning a zero food item will not raise blood sugar, and thus, maintain Ketosis. Inflammatory Factor (IF) is more complex, as it incorporates the Glycemic Load and many other factors, but it is a good indicator of the foods you should strive for in your diet, whether trying to lose weight or just eat healthy. Anything with positive IF number is good, or anti-inflammatory. Take a look at Tuna at 250; it's a super food. I suggest making it daily staple both on and off the diet. Nutritional Data also uses a statistic called Caloric Ratio, which is very similar to the PFC number that I use in HCG 2.0, but slightly more complex.

Nutritional Data then takes these statistics and ranks food items in several different categories such as fullness factor, weight loss, weight gain, optimal health and others. Let's look at a few examples. What you'll find is that NDs complex data roughly mirrors the simple PFC chart of proteins found in HCG 2.0.

Nutritional Data Food Graph Compared with P/FC of HCG 2.0

Food Item	eGL	IF	P/FC
Canned Tuna	0	250	31.1
Tilapia	0	21	11.8
Halibut	0	149	9.09
Bison (Sirloin)	0	34	8.92
Egg Whites	2	28	12.5
Chicken (breast)	0	-22	3.83
Beef (Sirloin)	0	2	2.83

As you can see, the items above coincide with the PFC chart we use in HCG 2.0. I invite you to visit NDs website for yourself. You'll also find that the protein items at the top of the PFC chart also rank very high in fullness factor, which gives you a greater feeling of satiety.

What is P/FC (PFC)? The PFC number is just a much simple way to calculate and rank your protein items. It's exactly what it says, the total protein in a food item divided by the total fat + total carbs. The higher the PFC number the better it is for you from a weight loss standpoint and there will always be a congruent relationship with a high PFC number and your portion sizes. If you want to eat a bigger meal select foods with a higher PFC number like Tuna. You'll also notice that most of the items with a high PFC number contain Omega 3 fats as opposed to Omega 6 fats. The calculation is listed below.

Protein ÷ (Fat + Carbs) = PFC

Protein
Fat + Carbs

> ➤ The PFC number will determine how much you can eat of a particular protein selection. The higher the number the larger the portion size. For example, for dinner you may have 100 grams (3.5 oz) of chicken breast which has 198 calories, or you may choose to have a whole 200 grams (7 oz) of Tilapia (192 calories). You decide.

> ➤ If your social schedule has prevented you from doing the diet in the past, HCG 2.0 has plenty of option for you. Depending on your BMR, a spinach and egg white omelet for breakfast and a tuna fish lunch could stockpile you 500-600 calories for a nice low-carb dinner.

Protein is the central focus of HCG 2.0. Protein is necessary to maintain lean muscle. Protein has no impact on ketosis. Protein provides the greatest effect on satiety, giving you a feeling of fullness. Most importantly protein is what makes a meal a meal, not only from a nutritional standpoint, but from a psychological and sociological standpoint as well. On any menu, protein is the main course; everything else is a side. Protein is the reason we were able to come down out of the trees and walk upright. Protein has given us the ability to think and reason. A meal without protein is merely a snack.

With this in mind, protein is our only caloric consideration on the HCG 2.0 diet. There are no overt starches or carbs allowed and fat is a by-product of our protein consumption as indicated by the graph below. The allowable calories on the HCG 2.0 diet are 40% of your BMR, Basal Metabolic Rate, which will be consistent with the protein allowed on the maintenance phase. What is BMR? Your BMR is the amount of calories you need on a daily basis to maintain normal, at rest, body function. These are the calories you need to keep your heart beating, your kidneys filtering, your lungs oxygenating and your brain thinking. This is why we use the BMR calculation to determine your specific caloric intake.

One of the biggest disconnects I found with the original HCG diet was that there were a fixed number of calories and protein across the board for all dieters. It alarmed me from the very beginning and after working with the diet for several years, it's still alarming. Not so much in the amount of calories, which is obviously very small, but more in its application to all dieters. This was an immediate red flag. I understand Dr. Simeons' theory that by supplementing HCG, additional calories will be obtained from abnormal fat, but to restrict each and every dieter- from big man to small woman- to the same caloric intake, specifically protein, seemed unreasonable. Not only will bigger people with greater muscle mass require more calories, specifically protein, they'll also have a diminished return on the calories being consumed from the perspective of satiety, which would make the diet considerably more difficult.

I quickly want to make one more point about protein. We're all aware that protein is what builds muscle, but a much overlooked function of protein is that amino acids, the building blocks of protein, are responsible for synthesizing neurotransmitters. These chemical messengers within the brain and nervous system play an important function in regulating mood. Many doctors believe that amino acid therapy can be as effective as traditional drugs used to treat anxiety and depression. These drugs are nearly as widespread as Aspirin these days and quite possible a result of inadequate amounts of protein in the SAD diet.

BMR Calculator: At this point, you're probably asking yourself how can you determine your BMR. Use the formula below to determine your BMR. You can also find a BMR calculator on my website, www.InsideOutWellness.net.

BMR Calculator for WOMEN

_64_ multiplied by 4.7 = _300.8_
Height (inches)   (A)

_141_ multiplied by 4.35 = _613.35_
Weight   (B)

_65_ multiplied by 4.7 = _305.5_
Age   (C)

_300.8_ + _613.35_ − _305.5_ + 655 = | _1263.65_ |
(A)   (B)   (C)   Your BMR

_1263.65_ multiplied by 0.40 = _505.46_

Your BMR   CALORIES ALLOWED ON LOW CALORIE DIET

BMR Calculator for MEN

_____ multiplied by 12.7 = _____
Height (inches)   (A)

_____ multiplied by 6.23= _____
Weight   (B)

_____ multiplied by 6.8 = _____
Age   (C)

—_____ + _____ − _____ + 66 = | |
(B)   (B)   (C)   Your BMR

_____ multiplied by 0.40 = _____

Your BMR   CALORIES ALLOWED ON LOW CALORIE DIET

Low Calorie Phase

1. Total allowable calories = BMR × 0.4 (Maximum of 1000 calories per day).

   ➢ All calories will be derived from a protein source listed from best to adequate in the graph on page 40. Each protein source has a P/FC number, which is the total ratio of protein in grams divided by fat plus carbs in grams.

2. I can't exactly say that vegetables are unlimited on HCG 2.0, but in the same breath, I dare you to overeat on veggies. They contain a lot of water and are therefore very filling. The more veggies you're consuming the less room you'll have for higher calorie, lower nutrient fillers. Calories from veggies DO NOT have to be subtracted from your total allowable calories. You need only keep your carb count below 30 grams per day.

   ➢ Use your veggie chart to select vegetable items that are lower in carbs. Green leafy vegetables are best. Carbs are your enemy on any Ketosis Diet and to maintain it you should strive to keep your carbs under 30 grams per day. I hate to limit the amount of veggies one can consume on any diet, but the fact of the matter is that carbs inhibit Ketosis. Even with the assistance of HCG its best to keep them below 30 grams per day for best results.

3. Of the allowable protein, do your best to get 15 to 20 grams of protein within 30 minutes of starting your day. This jump starts your metabolism, facilitating weight loss, with muscle maintaining protein. When you begin maintenance, men should strive for 30 grams and women 20 grams within the first 30 min.

4. The remainder of protein should be consumed with lunch and dinner, or even better, spread throughout the day in several small meals. The concept of breakfast, lunch and dinner is your boss's idea, not human physiology. It's best to eat smaller portions throughout the day like our hunter/gatherer ancestors.

5. Protein options are listed from best to adequate. Proteins with a higher P/FC number, i.e. tuna, are best known to induce and maintain Ketosis. Food items with a number of 3 or less don't necessarily have to be avoided, but your portion sizes are likely to be smaller. This is where you can use your own best judgment. Find a balance of what works best for you and your lifestyle. You have plenty of options.

6. There are no fruits, starches or sugar allowed.

Protein Chart (P/FC)

Food (100 g serving unless noted) 100 g = 3.5 oz	Calories	Protein (g)	Fat (g)	Carbs (g)	P/FC
Light Tuna (Canned in water)*	116	25.51	0.82	0	31.11
Mahi Mahi	85	18.5	0.7	0	26.43
Tuna Steak (Ahi)	130	22	1.5	0	14.67
3 egg whites	51	11.3	0.18	0.75	12.15
Tilapia*	96	20.08	1.7	0	11.81
Crab*	101	20.03	1.76	0	11.38
Lobster*	97	20.33	0.58	1.27	10.99
Halibut*	110	20.81	2.29	0	9.09
Bison (Sirloin)	113	21.4	2.4	0	8.92
Shrimp*	144	27.59	1.24	2.35	7.69
Non-fat cottage cheese	85	17.27	0.42	1.85	7.61
Cod*	122	20.91	3.59	0.41	5.23
Flounder*	133	22	4.24	0.41	4.73
Turkey Breast	187	28.7	7.2	0	3.99
Chicken (white meat)*	195	29.55	7.72	0	3.83
Pork Loin (4 oz)	154	23.29	6.13	0	3.80
Salmon	146	21.62	5.93	0	3.65
1% low fat cottage cheese	72	12.39	1.02	2.72	3.31
Whey Protein shake	170	30	2.5	7	3.16
1 oz beef jerky (zero carb variety)	60	11.2	4	0	2.80
Veal*	229	29.85	11.3	0	2.64
Trout	188	24.37	9.16	0.41	2.55
2% cottage cheese	90	13.74	1.93	3.63	2.47
Chicken (dark meat)	207	25.72	10.79	0	2.38
Beef Sirloin (lean)*	250	30.68	13.16	0	2.33
Pork Chop (1 Small Grilled)	118	13.12	6.85	0	1.92
Boca Meatless Burger (1)	90	15	2	6	1.88
Ground Beef (lean)*	248	25.71	15.35	0	1.67
1 serving container Greek Yogurt	130	17	3.5	7	1.62
Tofu (1/4 block)	88	9.37	5.54	2.18	1.21
1 whole egg	74	6.29	4.97	0.38	1.18
Ground Bison	223	18.67	15.93	0	1.17
Soy Protein Shake (1 pkg.)	120	14	2	14	0.88
Scallops	217	18.14	10.96	10.49	0.85
Catfish	240	17.57	14.53	8.54	0.76
Crimini Mushrooms	23	2	0	4	0.50
Sunflower Seeds (1/4 cup)	190	9	15	5	0.45
Lentils	353	25.8	1	60	0.42
Peanuts (1 oz)	161	7.31	13.96	4.57	0.39
Black beans	93	6	0.29	16.56	0.36
Navy beans	80	6	0	17	0.35
Dry Roasted Almonds (1 oz)	169	6.26	14.98	5.47	0.31
Dry Roasted Pistachios (1 oz)	161	6.05	13.03	7.59	0.29

The bulleted items below refer to the protein chart on page 40.

➢ All items on the traditional HCG diet are followed with an *.

➢ If you're curious about a particular protein item that isn't listed, simply calculate for yourself. Items with a number greater than 3 will be your best options.

➢ I included mushrooms in both the protein and vegetable chart. They're very low in calories, but they can really dress up your protein choice, more so than traditional veggies. They're also very rich in micronutrients, especially selenium.

➢ If you have a busy schedule, a Whey or Soy Protein shake can provide for a quick breakfast or lunch, but mind the carbs. Search for a product with highest amount of protein compared to the lowest amount of carbs. A good product will have a PFC greater than 3.

Vegetable Chart
Ranked from lowest in carbs to highest in carbs

Food (1 cup serving unless noted)	Calories	Protein (g)	Fat (g)	Carbs (g)
Pickles (Kosher)	5	0	0	1
Spinach*	7	0.86	0.12	1.09
Chard*	7	0.65	0.07	1.35
Lettuce*	8	0.5	0.08	1.63
Beet greens*	8	0.84	0.05	1.65
Celery*	14	0.7	0.17	3
Cucumbers*	16	0.68	0.12	3.6
Radishes*	19	0.79	0.12	3.94
Crimini Mushroom	23	2	0	4
Zucchini	20	1.5	0.22	4.15
Tomato (1 Med whole)*	22	1.08	0.25	4.82
Cabbage*	21	1.28	0.11	4.97
Asparagus*	27	3	0.16	5.2
Cauliflower	25	2	0.1	5.3
Broccoli	31	2.57	0.34	6
Bell Pepper (1 Med)	31	1	0.36	7.18
Squash	18	1.37	4.24	7.81
Brussel Sprouts	38	3	0.25	8
Fennel*	25	1	5.5	8.57
Edamame	110	8	3	10
Carrots	52	1.2	0.3	12.3
Onion*	67	1.47	0.13	16.18
Avocado (1 whole)	322	4.02	29.47	17.15

➢ All items on the traditional HCG diet are followed with an *.

➢ As you can see, there is not much variation among vegetable choices. When picking vegetables use the carb number as your best indicator, the lower the better, and **try to keep your carbs below 30 grams per day**.

➢ You'll notice that veggies with seeds on the inside and root vegetables (carrots, onions, etc.) will be higher in carbs. These are good and healthy food items, but higher carbs will slow Ketosis and thus should be limited on the low calorie phase of the diet.

➢ You may mix your vegetables.

Breakfast: 3 egg white omelet (51 cal) with spinach (1/2 cup) and tomatoes (1/2)

Lunch: Tuna Lettuce Wraps w/ Dill Pickle Relish (100 g. equals roughly one can drained) (116 cal)

> ➤ Add whatever veggies to tuna salad you want. By dicing, chewing and digesting them, the caloric intake is not relevant.
> ➤ Spinach Salad (2 cups, tomato 1/2, cucumber ½)
>   - ○ Use MCT oil or better yet, zero-calorie/carb alternative. Even better still, just use balsamic vinegar, salt and pepper.

Snack: 1 oz. beef zero-carb jerky (60 cal) 1 cup chicken bouillon (5 cal)

Dinner: Chicken Breast (150 grams or 5.25oz) w/sautéed peppers (245 cal) and steamed broccoli

Snack before bed: ½ serving whey protein shake (85 cal)

   - ○ You've probably been told not to eat before bed, but lean protein is good for you and will help you sleep. Most cellular repair and maintenance occur while you sleep. A lean protein source will feed this. You'll also rest better with calories in your system. Again, this is primitive hunter/gatherer physiology at work. When we're deprived of calories, the brain actually becomes more alert. It's looking for a food source. That's why you feel like laying your head down and taking a nap after lunch. Your brain is content with calories. A half serving of your protein shake will help you sleep and provide you with the proper nutrients for cellular repair and maintenance. A better evening snack would be something lower in carbs. Maybe a can of tuna with some celery sticks. I went with the protein shake to demonstrate that there are options if you have a sweet tooth.

Total Calories from Sample Day Above

Food Item	Protein (in grams)	Carbs (in grams)	Calories
3 egg whites	11.4	.75	51
Tuna (1 can)	25.5	0	116
Chicken (5.25oz)	45	0	292
Protein Shake (½)	15	3.5	85
Beef Jerky (1oz)	11.2	0	60
Total	108	4.25	604

> ➤ *If you wanted a larger dinner, what would happen to your portion size if you substituted the chicken breast for a Mahi Mahi Steak? You could actually consume a 12oz. Mahi Mahi Steak as an alternative to 5.25oz. of chicken breast. That's a lot of Mahi Mahi.*

> ➤ *I didn't list the fat content because it is a by-product of your protein and if you keep your 1:1 ratio of Omega 3s to 6s, it's of little concern.*

> ➤ *Nor did I count the calories from veggies. No need. Limit your carbs to fewer than 30 grams per day and there is no need to count calories from veggies. If we tallied all the carbs from the tomato, cucumber, broccoli and peppers, you'd be between 15 and 20 grams for the day, even including the protein shake before bed.*

> ➤ *I also chose to eliminate the calories from the MCT oil in your salad dressing (approximately 1 tablespoon per meal), because of its fat burning properties. Also, because there are plenty of zero-calorie/carb alternatives. Experiment for yourself. I've had patients use hot sauce, soy sauce, Sriracha, all sorts of things. The point here is if adding 100 calories per meal in salad dressing will be enough to motivate you to stay on the diet to completion, then by all means, add it. The goal of HCG 2.0 is a combination of weight loss and sustainability. **There is no failure: only variations of success.***

What you see above is a standard HCG 2.0 daily menu for a 5'6" woman trying to lose 25 pounds. It's not at all unreasonable, is it? It may not contain all of your favorites, but this is realistically how you should eat. Keep in mind that taste is an acquired sense. The more you get used to eating healthy, the more you'll like eating healthy. Once you shed the weight, which will happen quickly, you can begin to add the foods you love in moderation. With that said, you should take the 30-40 days of dieting to examine the foods you were eating prior that facilitated your weight gain. Were the poor foods you were eating a product of convenience? Habit? A busy social life? These are things you absolutely have to consider if you want to maintain your weight loss. Think of it in terms of positive and negative calories. What are positive and negative calories? It's nothing you'll find in a research journal, in fact, there is nothing scientific about positive and negative calories at all. It's something I made up, but it makes sense. It's a matter of necessity vs. luxury. Decide for yourself.

Positive Calories vs. Negative Calories – The difference is simple, the calories that provide you with sustenance are positive calories, and those that provide pleasure or taste are generally negative. The goal is to find a balance, and I'm speaking here from a perspective of lifestyle, not the HCG 2.0 diet. For example, you're not going to order your pizza without cheese. That would be foolish, but eliminating sausage or pepperoni and replacing with veggies will save you 100 calories. Or, do you really need to add a piece of cheese to your burger or your salad? The burger is positive; the cheese is negative, same with the salad. See where I'm going with this? Humans are habitual creatures, all of us. Many of your eating habits are exactly that... habits. Break them! Even just tweaking them a bit can easily reduce your caloric intake by 200-300 calories per day. Reducing dairy is a great way to start. Unless you're an infant, dairy can be completely eliminated from your diet... if you want it to be? There are so many examples of this that it's impossible to list them all. Examine your lifestyle and you'll soon find them for yourself. Find that balance between necessity and luxury.

Transition into the Low Calorie Phase

As you transition into the low calorie phase, it's important to note that it's not uncommon to experience hunger during the first week of the diet, peaking between days 5-7. This is because by day 4 and 5 you don't have the immediate calorie reserves from your loading and the HCG hasn't really began working for you at this early stage. With any hormone therapy, effects are cumulative and therefore not immediately apparent. After day 6 and 7 you should begin to experience the appetite suppressing effects of the HCG. Once this begins, the diet gets considerably easier. In fact, many report that they have difficulty eating all the allowable calories on the diet.

If you're accustomed to a high sugar diet consisting of soda, sugary snacks and/or high amounts of processed sugars, such as high fructose corn syrup, you may experience difficulty caused by de-toxing your body from these sugars. The most common symptoms are lightheadedness, headaches, fatigue and muscle-cramping. If you find these symptoms present get to a seated position and drink water. If they persist, call your doctor and in an emergency, call 911. There are supplements available to remedy these conditions which are discussed later.

Compare and Contrast Chart

Dr. Simeons' HCG Protocol	HCG 2.0 Protocol
Loading days focus on fatty foods and sugars (carbs).	Loading days focus on fatty foods with more emphasis on Omega 3 fats and fewer carbs.
Very Low Calorie Phase (VLCD) allows 500 calories for each person.	Low Calorie Phase is individualized, using one's BMR to calculate allowed calories. (Calories = 40% of BMR. All calories are derived from lean protein source utilizing P/FC number)
VLCD includes carbs, like melba toast and some fruits.	Low Calorie Phase emphasis is lean proteins with limited carbs and NO fruit.
VLCD doesn't allow food for breakfast, only coffee or tea.	Low Calorie Phase recommends the dieter eat a high protein, low calorie breakfast within 30 minutes of waking up (15-20 grams).
VLCD restricts proteins to only chicken, white fish, lean beef.	Proteins are ranked by PFC number. This number is used to determine portion sizes. The higher the number the better allowing for larger portions and more options.
VLCD is strict about eating only certain vegetables and not mixing them.	Low Calorie Phase allows unlimited vegetables, mixed if desired, as long as total carbs for the day remains under 30.
VLCD does not allow dieter to use certain skin products, shampoos, and cosmetics.	Low Calorie Phase has no restrictions on any of these types of products.
Dieter weighs him/herself every day.	Its recommended dieter weigh in only once per week.
Exercise is not allowed on traditional HCG diet.	Dieter should continue the same amount of exercise as they were doing prior to starting HCG 2.0. Also consider 20-30 min of walking before breakfast.
Limited choices for food and drink on the VLCD.	New food and drink items (like Crystal Light and protein shakes) give the dieter more options to keep them motivated and accommodate for a busier lifestyle. Any zero calorie/zero carb drinks are allowed.

Quick Summary of HCG 2.0

➢ BMR × 0.4 = Total Allowable Calories (All from protein).
  ✓ See chart on page 40 for best options

➢ Limit carbs to fewer than 30 grams per day. Budget them appropriately. If you need to have a protein shake for breakfast, you may have to limit carbs from veggies throughout the day.

  ✓ You might have "bad days." Try not to put them together consecutively, but if you do, DON'T GIVE UP!!!

Phase 3: Maintenance

Dr. Simeons has little to say regarding what to eat following your low calorie diet other than be cautious with sugar and starches, so this phase is largely up to interpretation. If you've completed the HCG diet plan with success, the last thing you want to do is waste all of your hard work and perseverance by immediately resorting to old eating habits. The first 3 weeks following the low calorie phase are absolutely critical to maintaining your weight loss. This cannot be stressed enough. Don't waste all your hard work by immediately resorting to old eating habits. **There are two things you need to understand before beginning maintenance.**

1. **Your body is not accustomed to its new weight**. Take a second and ask yourself how long it's been since you've been the weight you're currently at following the low calorie phase. Months? Years? Decades? As a result, your body will be determined to restore its fat reserves and return to your old, heavier weight that it is accustomed. Again, remember what Dr. Friedoff says, "The more weight you'd like to permanently lose, the more of your lifestyle you'll need to permanently change." HCG will certainly help you maintain your weight loss, but it cannot be unrealistically relied upon. If you're asking whether you'll gain the weight back, the answer is up to you and how closely you follow the maintenance recommendations below. The decision you make following your diet will determine your sustained weight loss.

2. **Taste is an acquired sense**. I say it every day in my office, and I've said it at least 3 times thus far. The longer you stay away from the poor foods that are often NOT your foods of choice, but rather your foods of convenience, the less you'll crave them. Likewise, the longer you expose yourself to healthy foods and vegetables, the better they'll taste. Keep this in mind when preparing meals for your young children.

Immediately following completion of your protocol, it's best to continue on the low calorie phase for three days after you discontinue your HCG supplement. During the first three weeks of maintenance you'll still want to stay away from carbs and sugar. It's during these first three weeks that your body will be most determined to replenish its fat stores and return to its old weight. Avoiding carbs is the best way to prevent this. You may begin to add dairy back into your diet, but carbs are your enemy during these first three weeks.

No More "Dieting"

After you lose the weight, the real "diet" begins

I say this to my patients on a daily basis. Unless you plan on doing another cycle of HCG, there is no more "dieting." The word "diet" has mistakenly assumed a short term connotation, when, in fact, your "diet" is your lifestyle. It's a culmination of all the food and drink you consume all day, every day. This is what you need to evaluate if you want to make your weight loss permanent. On a typical day, your "diet" should amount to roughly 125% of your BMR consisting of 40% protein, 40% fats (with a 1:1 ratio of Omega 3s to Omega 6s) and 20% carbs. Ideally, ALL of the carbs should come from fruit or root vegetables.

Keep in mind that these ratios are an aggregate. They may vary from day to day. For example, you may have a large pasta meal (using whole grain pasta, of course) one night, which will give you 400-500 calories in carbs, well over your allowable daily amount. This is ok, but the next day you'll have to limit your carbs to zero. Your new "diet" should provide you with a lifestyle you can both enjoy and realistically sustain. Let me say that again; your new "diet" should provide you with a lifestyle you can both enjoy and realistically sustain. All you have to do is eat smart and allocate the necessary amount of time to do so.

Counting Calories/Carbs

I know that counting calories and carbs can be tedious and even annoying to others at the dinner table, but it's important to know the rules and practice them until you can find a baseline for what works for you. This could take weeks or months or you might immediately be comfortable with your new weight and know exactly what you can eat and in what amounts to maintain it. This is where you'll need to educate yourself with the tools provided below. You may also want to consider the free smart phone app or website called My Fitness Pal. In addition to it having tremendous functionality as a calorie counter/converter, it also has a bar code reader that can tell you the calorie content and nutritional breakdown of nearly every food product on the planet, including restaurant items, bottled beverages and alcohol.

With that being said, for educational purposes, a calorie is a unit of energy. For simplicity, let's just say that calories are needed to provide energy so the body functions properly. The number of calories in a food is determined by the amount of energy the food provides. The number of calories a person needs depends on age, height, weight, gender, and activity level. All of these things combined are your BMR. The most accurate way to determine your BMR is through Bio-Impedance Analysis. More generically, but still very accurately, it can be calculated by using your height, weight and gender, which we provided you with earlier.

How to Maintain Your Weight Loss

To successfully maintain your weight loss, the amount of calories you'll consume on a daily basis will be determined by your new BMR. Your BMR will have to be recalculated given your new, reduced weight. In losing 20-30 pounds you BMR may have dropped by 100 to 200 calories. After finding your new BMR, you'll multiply it by 1.25 to give you your daily allowable calories. This is also the same calculation used by My Fitness Pal. Let's look at an example...

Gina is a 38 year old woman who lost 25 pounds on the HCG diet. Her new weight is 140 pounds. This makes her BMR 1364 calories.

1364 calories × 1.25 = 1705 calories per day.

1524.56

➢ *If Gina wants to maintain her new weight, she can consume up to 1705 calories per day, broken down into the following proportions...*

609

40% Protein - This will come primarily from meats, soy, nuts, lentils and a variety of other sources. There isn't nearly enough protein in the SAD as will be discussed.

609

40% Fats *w/ 1:1 ratio of Omega 3s to Omega 6s* - Omega 6's are the bad fats that clog your arteries, such as bacon, red meat, and dairy. The Omega 3s are good fats necessary for the body to make cellular membranes, steroid hormones and good cholesterols. Examples of good Omega 3s are fish, avocado and nuts. This doesn't have to be a precise calculation, but, as an example, if you have bacon and eggs for breakfast, you should have tuna and avocado for lunch. Strive for balance.

- With the exception of dairy, avocado, oils, nuts and salad dressing, most of your fat consumption will be a by-product of your protein. If you stick with protein choices high on the PFC list, you'll only have to worry about excessive amounts of dairy when calculating your calories from fat, as avocado and nuts, both Omega 3s, are of the good fat variety. If you're curious, biochemists don't just make up names for these things. The term Omega 3 has to do with the double bonding of carbon that occurs at the 3rd carbon from the end of a long-chain fatty acid. This is called the Omega carbon as opposed to the Alpha carbon at the beginning.

304.91

20% Carbs - It would be best to get all of these from fruit or root vegetables (sweet potatoes, onions, carrots, etc.), but I know that might be unrealistic. Just do your best to stay away from everything white, which, as a general rule, is a bench mark for how processed a food item is to be. Highly refined carbohydrates and sugars are so rapidly digested that the rush of incoming fuel cannot be fully metabolized and these calories ultimately end up stored as fat. If there is a single piece of information that you take away from this book, it should be to eliminate processed carbs and sugar from your diet. Stick to whole grain pastas and wheat bread... or just eat more protein and vegetables.

- I'd be ignoring the elephant in the room if I didn't mention alcohol. As is life, moderation is the key. Not only is alcohol extremely high in calories (7 calories per gram), over-consumption can be taxing on the liver. If your liver is busy oxidizing alcohol, it's not oxidizing fats which then accumulate both in the liver (fatty liver disease) and systemically. Beer and wine is going to be highest in calories followed by straight liquors. Definitely avoid sugary mixers that can double and even triple the caloric intake. Mix with water or diet soda... in moderation.

- *Unlimited vegetables are allowed during maintenance. Steam them for best nutritional value.*

Let's take another look at our example to find out how many calories in protein, fat and carbs Gina can consume on a daily basis.

1705 total calories × 0.4 protein = 682 calories from protein

1705 total calories × 0.4 fat = 682 calories from fat (341 from Omega 6s and 341 from Omega 3s)

1705 total calories × 0.2 carbs = 341 calories from carbs w/most from fruit and root veggies

➤ Use protein and veggie chart to maximize your portion sizes.

What you see above is an entirely reasonable amount of calories. As an example, in a single day, Gina could have 3 eggs, 2 cans of tuna, a 10 oz. bison steak, , a sweet potato with a table spoon of real butter, an apple, 3 oz of beef jerky and all the veggies her healthy heart desires and still have a couple hundred calories to spare. How amazing is that? Or, she could have one McDonalds Big Mac meal and a medium milkshake. Yes, the caloric values are the same, but the latter provides you with next to zero nutritional value. Nobody really wants to eat McDonalds, but it's convenient. Make the time to eat healthy. IT WILL SAVE YOUR LIFE!

Again, these numbers are an aggregate. If Gina wants to have pasta and a couple of glasses of wine on a Friday night, resulting in a carb intake of 600 calories, she can certainly do that if she limits her carbs on Thursday and Saturday. This is a trial and error process, but until you become comfortable with what works for you, it's best to error on the side of caution.

More Comparing and Contrasting

The glaring difference between HCG 2.0 and the traditional diet is the elimination of fruit and bread sticks which is replaced by lean protein. A greater understanding of food chemistry provides a ranking system of your protein that allow for larger portion sizes of items with higher protein to calorie ratio, which is reflected in the PFC. Not only does this facilitate greater Ketosis and weight loss, but protein provides a greater satiety effect than fruit. Protein, as compared to fruit, also gives you the ceremonial effect of a meal that fruit just doesn't provide. What I mean by this is there is a lot to be said about the act of sitting down and having a meal. This is a dwindling tradition in America. We often eat in our cars or on the run and consume as many calories as possible in a minimal amount of time. Not only is the omnivorous diet of humans not designed for this behavior, but it takes the fun out of eating. Find time to sit down and enjoy your food. All these little things that are taken for granted could be the difference in maintaining your weight loss.

Other minor differences are the inclusion of new food items such as zero calorie, zero carb drinks and whey or soy protein shakes. You might notice that HCG 2.0 is not all that different from the South Beach Diet, The Dukan Diet, The Paleo Diet, or other Ketosis Diets. The reason is because Ketosis works and is best achieved with the elimination of carbs, all the time. **Ketosis is the door to unlocking stored fat, HCG is the key.**

A Word for the Critics

I'd be overlooking a common criticism of HCG if I didn't address its detractors that suggest it is merely a placebo. It's true; most of the research on HCG dates back to the 50s, 60s, and early 70s and is mostly clinical. However, there was a small study recently published in The Bariatrician, a medical journal published by the American Society of Bariatric Physicians. The study offered more evidence that HCG works. Subjects placed on the HCG diet lost 30% more weight than counterparts who were put on a conventional meal replacement plan, but regardless, a lack of evidence doesn't disprove. Additionally, you can't discredit the positive results seen by millions that have used HCG with success. This was echoed by Dr. Oz when HCG was featured on his show in 2011, and recapped in First for Women Magazine, "Sometimes the experience of real people doesn't agree with science. And sometimes it's because the science hasn't caught up. When we see real people do things that work, we in the medical field have to pay attention."

With or without an overwhelming amount of evidence, the point I'd like to make is that if you're questioning the placebo effects of HCG, you're missing the bigger picture. The fact is; HCG dieters lose a lot of weight, typically 20-30 pounds, in just 30-40 days. If this is the desired effect, whether HCG is entirely or just partially responsible, you have to ask yourself, does it really matter? A controlled study would certainly answer a lot of questions, but until then, we'll have to persevere with the research we have. For those who dismiss the reality of it, the secret will be safe with us.

Coincidentally, what you'll find is that the biggest critics of HCG weight loss are from those individuals that have never struggled with their weight. These people are of the simple belief that if you eat too much, you get fat, and if you want to lose weight, it's merely a matter of eating less. Don't let the likes of these dissuade you. You'll have last word, trust me.

Something I like to make my patients aware of, maybe to my detriment, is that there is a placebo effect in all of medicine. Voltaire said it best, "the art of medicine is doctor entertaining patient while nature takes its course." The act of being proactive with your health is a placebo in and of itself. Look at it this way… I pay $85/per month for my gym membership. I hate going to the gym. I could get the same workout in my basement with some dumb bells, a Swiss ball and pair of jogging shoes. I'm aware of it, yet I continue to pay the $85 every month because it forces me to commit and that makes it worth it. The act of showing up and allocating 45 minutes, 3-4 times per week to get the physical activity I need to maintain a healthy weight and my desired aesthetic appearance is worth the $85. The same can be said of dieters; a financial commitment drives success. In exchange for the money we spend, we want a very specific set of rules to guide our behavior, which, more frequently than not, will lead to positive results. The placebo is not in the HCG, but in being proactive with your health; making that initial commitment, whether financial or otherwise, is the first step in this process.

Getting Started

Before You Begin Your Diet

Over the next couple of sections, we'll discuss recommendations that have been beneficial to my patients.

First and foremost, you'll want to find a good HCG product, whether it be prescribed from a physician or the non-prescription homeopathic drops. I work with both in my practice and both are effective under the right circumstances. If you're new to HCG weight loss, the gauntlet of information on the internet can be a challenge to navigate, but, over the next few pages, I'll do my best to answer all of your questions regarding the type of HCG product that is right for you.

As a general rule, I typically have patients start with the non-prescription drops. They're affordable and effective. If you have a significant amount of weigh to lose and you plan on doing multiple rounds of the diet, you may want to try a mix of the homeopathic and the prescription, not at the same time, but alternating between the two from one round of the diet to the next. This limits the tolerance you can develop for one product or the other and maintains consistent weight loss. This has been very successful for my patients that are 300 to 400 pounds and up. Some of these patients have been gracious enough to journal about their weight loss and post their entries to my blog. See for yourself, it can be very inspirational.

What You Need to Know Before You Purchase

What you need to know is that there are two main variations on HCG products; prescription and non-prescription, which is also known as homeopathic. This alone is simple enough, but the confusion is in the delivery mechanism or the process in which you consume the HCG. Hormones are very large molecules. Because of their size, they're not readily absorbed through the GI like other medications that you simply swallow, so hormones are typically injected subcutaneously, the same way a diabetic would inject insulin. However, hormones can also be absorbed through the oral cavity. As a result, many pharmacies have been quick to make dissolvable products that are taken orally, like sublingual tablets and lozenges that are more patient-friendly. Both products are compared below.

Variations of HCG

Non-Prescription (Homeopathic)

Before discussing the drops, let's briefly define homeopathy. This alternative medical system was developed in Germany at the end of the 18th century. It is based on the "law of minimal dose" — with the focus being that exposure alone to a particular compound provides the greatest effect. The Homeopathic HCG that you'll find from an FDA approved manufacturer uses the intact HCG molecule, in combination with a magnification process, to increase its potency. You'll find this on the label under drug facts. The Homeopathic HCG used in my practice is labeled (3X, 6X, 12X, 30X, 60X), which is an indication of its potency. This may raise eyebrows, and I was skeptical at first too. In fact, it was only recently that I introduce the drops into my practice; prior to that I was working only with the prescription HCG. I did so as a result of overwhelming patient demand. I had so many requests for the drops because they'd had a friend or family member do so well with the product that they wanted to use it themselves. I spent months, wasting my breath, arguing with patients as to why the prescription product was better before I finally broke down and did some investigating. I soon found a FDA approved, homeopathic manufacturer that assured me his product would get equal, if not better results than the prescription HCG that I'd been using. I began recommending it as a more affordable alternative to the prescription HCG and was so impressed with the results that I now use it almost exclusively. It's been my experience that there is little difference in weight loss when comparing the homeopathic drops to prescription HCG. This is echoed by Linda Prinster, author of The HCG Weight Loss Cure Guide, which is used by many MDs as the patient education piece to accompany the diet. Prinster says that with committed patients both prescription and homeopathic HCG products will yield weight loss of 20-30 lbs. in 30-40 diet days. I included a graph from her book that compares and contrasts the Homeopathic, the injections and the sublingual, or what she refers to as mixed HCG, because of the mixing agent used to facilitate absorptions through the oral cavity.

There are some exceptions, usually when a patient gets closer to their goal weight, when the prescription product will be more effective. This usually occurs with patients that are struggling to lose that last 10 to 15 pounds. This pertains to dieters that have lost a considerable amount of weight and just can't shake that last 10 to 15, rather than those men or woman who put on a few pounds over the winter and are trying to get back into swimsuit shape. The non-prescription drops will work fine for the latter, but that last 10-15 can be difficult to shake for many. The reason is because the closer you get to your goal weight, the stingier your body will be with releasing its fat reserves, especially if you've been overweight for a long time. This is when a more concentrated HCG, like that of the prescription product, may be more effective. The downside here is the expense involved. The prescription product is often 3 to 4 times the cost; the reason being that it is usually compounded at a boutique type pharmacy and individualized to each patient.

My only warning regarding the non-prescription drops is that the quality can vary significantly. There are many internet retailers out there trying to make a quick buck on a hot industry. In December 2011, the US Federal Drug Association, and the Federal Trade Commission, issued warning letters to seven online retailers of homeopathic HCG. The letters warned that selling drugs unapproved by the FDA was illegal, in addition to making unsupported and exaggerated claims regarding HCG and its effects on weight loss. My advice here is to be careful with what you purchase via the Internet. I don't feel that there's any danger with purchasing a product online, but the quality could be suspect. If you're purchasing online, at the very least make a phone call to find out if the retailer has a medical professional on staff. Also, stay away from any HCG retailer that offers a guarantee. Medical professionals don't offer guarantees.

Injections - Injections were the method used by Dr. Simeons in his clinic. His dosages ranged from 125 IUs to 200 IUs. He warned that increasing dosages beyond those ranges could, in fact, be counter-productive, which may account for why the homeopathic version is equally as effective. During the time Dr. Simeon was practicing, prior to bio-identical hormones therapy, the HCG hormone was harvested from the urine of pregnant women, usually in underdeveloped countries, which made for an unsterile product. Many have concluded that this is why the diet disappeared for nearly 50 years, as a result of a Foot and Mouth epidemic that broke out in the UK from unsterile HCG. I can't say this with complete certainty, but I felt it worth mentioning. It seems logical that this could be the reason the diet lost popularity so quickly. Now days, with the advances in bio-identical hormone therapy, HCG is compounded in a pharmacy and mixed with bacteriostatic water. Bio-identical Hormone therapy uses a protein from a yam or soy bean and alters it to become the exact replica of that which is produced in the human body, creating a safe and sterile product. As I said earlier, it's typically made at compounding pharmacies that specialize in individualized medicine, but there are also brand name products such as Pregnyl and Organon. What you have to remember, is that a bio-identical hormone is the same regardless of where it's compounded. The reason I say this is to help you find the most affordable product. It's kind of like buying aspirin or ibuprofen; the molecular makeup is the same, regardless of the name brand, so save yourself a couple of bucks and buy generic.

Sublingual - As I stated above, when I began working with HCG, injections were the only available option. As the diet gained in popularity, pharmacies were quick to develop more patient-friendly HCG products that don't involve syringes. The sublingual tablet w/B12 is the most common, but there are also trans-dermal creams, lozenges and nasal sprays. The sublingual tablet is now the product of choice. Given the widespread availability of alternatives to the injections, and the recent fungal meningitis outbreak at the New England Compounding Center; I no longer work with injections, as they are unnecessarily invasive, especially for home use. Some patients are of the belief that by injecting themselves with a needle, the procedure is more therapeutic, and thus will lead to greater weight loss, but this is not true. The sublingual tablets are equally as effective. If you're still determined to do the injections, there are still plenty of practitioners prescribing them, but first see the advantages to the sublingual tablets below.

Advantages of Sub-Lingual Tablets Over Injections

1. The shelf-life of the HCG tablets is 12 months, compared to 60 days for the HCG injections.
2. The HCG tablets do not need to be refrigerated.
3. HCG tablets are easier to travel with.
4. HCG tablets are safer, as there is no risk of infection.
5. You don't have to stick yourself every day.

There will always be debate over which product is better, but my advice is start with the drops. They're affordable and effective. If you're not getting the desired results from one product or the other, you can always switch.

Below is a chart from Linda Prinster's book, *The HCG Weight Loss Cure Guide*. It does a good job of comparing and contrasting the different products. I also recommend discussing this with your doctor. However, be prepared for a questionable reaction. You may even have to educate them on the protocol. Most MDs, although very well-educated and altruistic, are indoctrinated to treat illness, rather than prevent it. Don't be dissuaded. Any weight loss plan, with the exception of amphetamine based diet pills, that involves the elimination of processed sugars and carbs, is good for you.

Compare and Contrast Chart **from Linda Prinster's The HCG Weight Loss Cure Guide**

	Type 1 **Homeopathic HCG** (Professional strength homeopathic remedy made in an FDA approved U.S. laboratory; no mixing required)	Type 2 **Injected HCG** (Prescription HCG mixed by you or pharmacist)	Type 3 **Sublingual, Mixed HCG** (Prescription HCG mixed with B12 or another mixing agent by you or pharmacist)
Taken	By mouth, under tongue; also referred to as sublingually	By Injection	By mouth, under tongue; also referred to as sublingually
Pain	None	Little to None	None
Taste	Almost Tasteless	None	Depends in mixing solution, i.e. B12 tastes like the liquid baby vitamins used in the 1970s
Time	4 minutes if taken 2 times per day; 6 minutes if taken 3 times a day	About 1 minute; once per day	4 minutes when taken 2 times per day
Fear	None	Usually none after the first time, but can be stressful	None
Typical Weight Loss per Cycle	With committed participants, 20-30 lbs. in 30-40 diet days	With committed participants, 20-30 lbs. in 30-40 diet days	With committed participants, 20-30 lbs. in 30-40 diet days

Exercise

Exercise was not recommended on the original diet, in fact, most patients were treated on an in-patient basis. My rule of thumb regarding exercise is do what you were doing prior to starting the diet. If you were not exercising prior to starting the diet, but committing to losing weight has inspired a new attitude towards health and fitness, as that which frequently happens in early January during New Year's Resolution Season, then walking for 30-45 minutes per day is a good place start. You'll want to walk at a brisk pace where your breathing becomes slightly strained to the point where talking becomes difficult. This is an ideal pace for weight loss.

Vigorous cardio such is jogging or spinning is not recommended nor is it conducive for weight loss. Your body is a lot smarter than you think and when you begin these vigorous cardio workouts, you actually become more efficient with your calories, which will work against your weight loss. This is a similar concept to "starvation mode." By increasing heart rate for long periods of time, your body assumes you're out chasing wild game across the prairie and will strive to maintain a calorie reserve. Burning off an excessive number of calories, as which occurs during rigorous cardio workouts, makes your body more determined to store away excess calories in fat. I'm in no way, shape or form discouraging heavy cardio workouts, but save them until after you lose the weight.

Ideal exercises to enhance weight loss

1. **Brisk walking** for 30-60 minutes per day. If possible, get 30 minutes prior to breakfast. I know, the numbers don't quite add up, but walking is the only exception to not getting your protein in the first 30 min of your day. Both the walking and the protein help to jumpstart your metabolism and enhance your Ketogenic Response. If you want to guarantee your success, this is the best way to do it from both a physiological and motivational perspective. If you start your day with motivation you'll likely finish it with motivation.

2. **Light-weight/high-repetition weight training** - You're not trying to build muscle, but burn fat. Cross fit is an example of this type of workout, but sometimes combines too much cardio. Cross fit is great to make routine after you complete the low-cal phase of the diet, but be cautious during the low cal phase, especially

if you have no experience. Again, you're not trying to build muscle, but burn fat. Save the muscle-building for after the diet.

3. **Isometric exercises** like Yoga, Pilates or Swiss Ball routines are excellent for maintaining muscle mass.

4. **Vibration Plate Workout** – Most gyms have vibration plates now and they're becoming increasingly more affordable for purchase in the home. These machines that vibrate at extremely high rates were developed by NASA to help astronauts in space maintain bone density in a weightless environment, but they were quickly found to have weight loss properties. Your brain has an innate desire to maintain stability. The shaking effect of the vibration plate causes your core musculature to fire constantly in an attempt to maintain balance and stability. You can get a high powered workout in just 10 minutes. I have one in my office and use it myself. There is more information on my blog regarding vibration plates.

5. **Commercial Workouts** – What are commercial workouts? These are recommendations I give to my pain management patients. When you're sitting in front of the TV in the evening, hop off the couch during the commercials and plank for a minute. I also have more information on my blog illustrating a variety of exercises you can do right in front of the TV.

➢ *All of these are best for converting fat mass to lean mass without extended periods of raised heart rate, which is ideal for weight loss.*

Things to Do Before Starting Diet

1. **Pick a start date** and tell your family and friends. Let them know that you'll soon be making some lifestyle changes as part your new outlook on your health. Not only will this ensure their support, but more importantly, it commits you to it. Better yet, find a friend or loved one to do the diet with you. As Deepak Chopra says, "success comes when people act together; failure tends to happen alone."

2. **Clean out your cabinets and refrigerator** of all the junk food items that might be filling it. This is an easy way to avoid temptation. This may be difficult if you have kids in the house, but it's also an opportunity to make improvements in their diet as well.

3. **Visit your Doctor** for a routine check-up and blood work. In addition to getting the green light from your physician to begin a weight loss program, you'll also be able to compare your pre and post diet metabolic panel. You might be surprised at what a 30-40 day cycle of the HCG diet can do to improve cholesterol, blood glucose, HBA1C and blood pressure. I've written several blogs about the positive effects I've seen HCG have on blood chemistry. Visit for yourself.

4. **Go to the grocery store**. You're investing in your health and appearance so spare no expense. Buy organic as these foods have a higher ratio of nutritional content to calories. Experiment with things you've never tried before. For recipe tips, visit my blog. I try to add something new and fun on a weekly basis.

5. **Prepare your food ahead of time.** Thaw out frozen meats. Grill some chicken breasts. Prepare some tuna salad. Cut and refrigerate vegetables. The poor foods we eat are seldom our foods of choice, but more often our foods of convenience. You're probably to the point that you can finish my sentences by now, but I can't say it enough; setting the alarm clock 15 minutes earlier in the morning to prepare your meals can make all the difference in your success.

    ➢   Again, this diet doesn't have to be the undertaking of a lifetime for you to achieve your desired results, but the recommendations above and below will help and motivate you.

Recommended Products to Accompany Diet

You don't have to spend an arm and a leg on additional products for the diet. The products below are recommended, but not required.

1. **MCT Oil** – MCT stands for medium-chain triglyceride. It's tasteless oil that is more readily absorbed by the GI than traditional oils. It's also been linked to promoting weight loss. Clinical studies published in the American Journal of Clinical Nutrition suggest that small changes in the quality of fat intake can be useful to enhance weight loss. MCT oil is best used to combine with Balsamic or Apple Cider Vinegar for a low calorie salad dressing. This is a better alternative to Olive Oil or store bought salad dressings. Better yet, just use vinegar alone with some additional salad seasoning. Or try adding soy sauce or hot sauce. Both of these are zero calorie/carb. Just because it's not the norm doesn't mean it isn't tasty. Call me crazy, but I love dipping celery in hot sauce. Try it.

2. **Stevia** – If you're a coffee or tea drinker and like it sweet, this is a must. Sweet Leaf is a good brand. Others may contain dextrose. Any unnecessary, negative calories should be eliminated at all costs. Calories from sugary beverages are the first place to start.

3. **Protein Replacement Shakes** – These are recommended if you have a busy schedule and don't have time to prepare your foods. Remember your PFC. A good protein shake should have a number greater than 3. This can be a good and convenient breakfast option to have after your 30 minute morning walk. Limit your carbs by doing half or a 2/3 serving.

4. **Chicken Broth or Bouillon** – This can be used to simmer meats or veggies, as an alternative to cooking oil and it can also be sipped as a snack to hold you over between meals. The sodium facilitates protein absorption.

5. **Beef Jerky** – This makes a great in-between meal snack. It has an adequate P/CF if you find the zero-carb variety, which will not inhibit Ketosis. You may have to purchase online or from a Whole Foods. I'm a big fan of Whole Foods, but it should more appropriately be called Whole Paycheck. Again, find a balance.

Recommended Supplements to Add to Diet Protocol

Let me start off by saying that supplements shouldn't be seen as a replacement, but rather a compliment to a healthy, whole food diet. The better your diet, the less you'll need in terms of vitamin supplementation. This doesn't mean you don't need supplements, but in the same breath, don't be fooled by every scare care ad you see on TV suggesting that if you don't take their particular product you'll end up in a wheel chair by age 50. There are a million different vitamin and herbal supplements on the market to support every body system and remedy every illness or condition imaginable, but nothing is as effective in maintaining your health as a healthy, whole food diet.

If you're unfamiliar, a whole food is a food that is unprocessed or unrefined. If you've ever heard someone tell you to shop the perimeters, the reason is because most of the whole foods are located on the perimeters. The stuff you'll find throughout the middle of the grocery store will be more processed and is manufactured for longer shelf life rather than your health. If you're like me and don't like going to the grocery store, shopping the perimeters is the way to go. Everything seems to flow around the perimeters, am I right? As soon as I venture into the middle for the one odd ball condiment I need, I suddenly turn into a tourist in a foreign country; I'm turning around in circles, trying to read signs, asking for directions... it's awful.

This is a good point for me to mention whole food supplements, which are a better alternative to your standard synthetic vitamin supplements you find at your local pharmacy. Whole food supplements are, like their name suggests, supplements made from concentrated whole foods, primarily fruits and vegetables. The vitamins found within these supplements are organic in nature and not isolated. They are highly complex and combine a variety of enzymes, coenzymes, antioxidants and activators all working together within the body.

Synthetic vitamins, like the ultra-high dose formulas mentioned above are isolated replications. Let's take Vitamin C for example. When you eat an orange, you're getting real Vitamin C. However, when you eat a chewable Vitamin C tablet, what you're actually getting is a synthetic version of Vitamin C called Ascorbic Acid. Although it's molecularly the same, the manufactured and isolated version of Vitamin C (Ascorbic Acid) is seen by the body as more of foreign substance and not absorbed and processed with the same efficiency as its organic counterpart. An easy way to determine whether a supplement is a whole food supplement is by looking at the label. A whole food supplement warrants a real food label like that you'd see on a carton of milk or food product. Synthetic labels look different and probably have dosages that are measured in International Units (IUs). Another way to determine the difference is by cost. The whole food supplements are probably 3-5 times the cost, although worth it.

1. **Multi-Vitamin** – Specifically a whole food supplement like I mentioned above. Juice Plus has a great product. In lieu of the fruit you won't be eating during the low calorie phase, this is highly recommended.

2. **Biotin** – This is recommended more for women than men and highly recommended for women that have any family history of female pattern baldness or who have lost hair following a pregnancy. Hair loss can be an adverse effect of HCG and biotin will help prevent this. I've seen this only once in my office. I find it worth mentioning that the woman, despite her hair loss, refused to quit the diet. She was having such great success that she said she'd rather be thin and bald, than overweight. I'm happy to say that all her hair grew back following her protocol.

3. **Potassium** – If you're taking a multi-vitamin it will likely have potassium, so you won't need to double up. This is especially recommended if you're used to eating a diet high in sugar. These patients may suffer muscle cramping and the Potassium can remedy this.

Steps to Avoid Hunger

With any diet or restriction in calories from a previous norm, you're going to experience some hunger. HCG is no different. However, with HCG your hunger pangs usually peak around days 5 and 6 and then quickly subside as the HCG begins to tap into your unwanted fat, converting it into calories.

So what do you do during days 5-7?

The good news is that while your hunger is peaking during the first week, so is your weight loss. The most exaggerated weight loss on the HCG diet is experienced in the first 10 days to two weeks. So while you're hungry and possibly frustrated during the first week, you're also being rewarded with losing 1-2 pounds per day. This will motivate you to continue knowing that your sacrifice is already paying off and the hunger will soon subside.

However, to help you make it through the first week, following the steps below can make the transition into the low calorie phase much easier.

1. **Load properly** - I know the loading days seem counter-productive, but this phase of the HCG diet is equally as important as the low-cal phase. Not only does proper loading provide an immediate calorie reserve to sustain you in days 3, 4 and 5, but the sudden increase in fat consumption sparks the metabolization of fat, thus jump-starting the diet. It also sidesteps "starvation mode," which we discussed earlier. So, over-consume on the fattiest foods you love. Carbs are okay too, but the focus should be fats. If this concerns you, over-consume on healthy Omega-3 fats like salmon, avocado and nuts. The bottom line, ask yourself what you can do to add more fat to your meals and do it.

2. **Prepare allowable foods ahead of time** - Preparing your meals ahead of time will help you avoid temptation when you find yourself vulnerable.

3. **"Cheat" Properly** – I put cheat in quotations because it's a word my patients use, not me. I've said it before, there is no cheating, only variations of success. If you have a couple of bad days, don't give up. By the end of your protocol you'll be down 20+ pounds.

    I often recommend a few food items to help patients sustain themselves in the first week of the diet, as I'd rather them "cheat" with foods that will have little or no impact on their success. They're listed below...

1. **Green Vegetables** – I know we said limit your carbs to under 30 grams per day, but if you must nibble, best to nibble on some veggies. Many green veggies have negative calories. The calories you burn by chewing and digesting are greater than that which is being consumed. Dress them up with balsamic vinegar or spices.

2. **Chicken Bouillon** - Most chicken bouillon cubes or pouches contain only 5-20 calories per serving, but sipping a cup can be quite filling. Add some spinach, green onions and an egg white and you've got a 40 calorie version of egg-drop soup. Don't be concerned about the sodium because the positive effect of weight loss is greater than negative effect of increased sodium consumption. Sodium also facilitates your protein absorption.

3. **Beef Jerky** - Not the crappy stuff you buy from a gas station, but quality, zero-carb, preferably organic, beef jerky that can be found at a Whole Foods or your local meat market. Beef jerky has a good P/FC ratio, making it a convenient and non-ketosis inhibiting snack food. An ounce or two in between your meals accompanied by a couple of celery stalks makes a great snack.

4. **Eat more protein** – Beef Jerky was suggested because of the convenience of it. If you're absolutely starving pick a high protein, low fat/carb item and have a snack. Tuna is a perfect for this. Add a table spoon of Dill Relish and wrap in a Romaine Leaf for a zero-carb snack. Be smart with your calories.

5. **Eat a piece of gum** – Or a **sip a sweet zero calorie/carb beverage**. The sweetness alone will be enough to get some insulin pumping. I know, many say these zero calorie beverages are not allowed, and I would agree that water and tea are better alternatives, but if you're one of those people that *need* a Diet Coke in the afternoon, then by all means do so. This is an example of one of the little things that can be a BIG roadblock for many would be dieters. Or, it could be the straw that broke the camel's back causing you to quit prematurely. The key is to find a balance. After you shed the weight, you can then address your Diet Coke habit. For your information, the sweetness alone, whether it's accompanied by calories or sugar, sparks the pancreas to release insulin. A secondary effect of insulin is appetite suppression.

6. **Brush your teeth** when hungry. This has been suggested by a couple of my patients. Give it a try.

Closing

I tell my pain management patients on a daily basis that only YOU can feel your pain, and only YOU can take the steps necessary to remedy it. Dieting is no different. The first step is the most difficult, but once you make the commitment to take control of your health and wellbeing, good things will most certainly follow. There is no failure on HCG 2.0, only variations of success!

1. What is HCG?
2. Is the HCG diet safe for men?
3. What are the positive effects of HCG?
4. What are some negative side effects sometimes experienced while HCG is present in the body?
5. What about homeopathic HCG?
6. How exactly does HCG allow you to lose weight?
7. Why the 500 calorie diet (VLCD very low calorie diet)?
8. How is the HCG protocol different from any other diet out there?
9. What will I eat on this protocol?_
10. How does this program compare to others?

What is HCG?

HCG (Human Chorionic Gonadatropin) is a hormone produced during pregnancy. The purpose of the HCG hormone is to rally the metabolism of systemic fat. Typically, as a species, the human body is pre-disposed to retain calories in the form of fat reserves as a survival mechanism for long winters or famine: conditions that rarely exist today. This is why dieting is such an uphill battle; not only are we struggling with our own poor eating habits, but a genetic predisposition to retain fat. **HCG is the solution**. When a woman becomes pregnant, the growing baby requires a 24/7 calorie source. In response, the placenta of the mother begins to produce HCG, which "unlocks" her stored fat to provide the calories necessary for proper development of her unborn child. If the HCG hormone is supplemented in the absence of a pregnancy, the dieter can sustain themselves on their own stored fat, resulting in healthy weight loss.

Is the HCG diet safe for Men?

Yes! The HCG protocol is safe for men. Men are often more uncomfortable with any sort of hormone therapy, which we tend to associate with sex or a deficiency in that department. This is echoed by Dr. Simeons, "It neither makes men grow breasts nor does it interfere with their virility, though where this was deficient it may improve it. It never makes women grow a beard or develop a gruff voice. I have stressed this point only for the sake of my lay readers, because, it is our daily experience that when patients hear the word hormone they immediately jump to the conclusion that this must have something to do with the sex- sphere."

Also keep in mind that ALL men were exposed to extremely high concentrations of HCG in the womb and most of us turned out ok, right? Men, in fact, generally have more success with the diet than women. While women typically lose .5 lb. - 1lb. per day, men typically lose 1 to 2 lbs per day.

What are the positive effects of HCG?

Besides the accelerated weight loss and body re-shaping, many patients report:

- Better rest.
- Improvements in blood chemistry including lowered cholesterols, blood pressure and HBa1C, which typically remains low following the diet.
- Higher energy levels without a nervous or edgy feeling.
- A general feeling of well-being.

What are the negative side effects?

While on the protocol a few patients report:

- Headaches early in the protocol. This could be more of problem if you are accustomed to a high sugar diet and more likely a by-product of detoxing yourself than the HCG. This can be addressed with Aspirin.
- Leg cramping. Again, this is typically a more frequent problem if you were accustomed to a high sugar diet. A multi-vitamin or potassium supplement can help remedy this.
- Slight, temporary hair thinning, primarily in women. You may be more likely to experience this if you have a history of female pattern baldness of have lost hair following a pregnancy. A Biotin supplement can remedy this.

What is homeopathic HCG?

Homeopathic HCG comes in a liquid and is taken sublingually (under your tongue). It's an affordable but effective alternative to prescription HCG. It's recommended that it is purchased from a health care provider.

How exactly does HCG allow you to lose weight?

This is best answered by relating HCG to its function during pregnancy. HCG is produced by the placenta of pregnant women with the sole purpose of providing a 24/7 calorie source for the growing baby. It does so by tapping into fat stores in our bellies, arms and thighs, releasing those calories to be used as an energy source for the growing baby. In the absence of a pregnancy the hormone can supplemented to produce the same effect, putting 1500 to 4000 calories per day of stored fat into the system, allowing the dieter to sustain themselves on their own stored fat - resulting in rapid, but healthy fat loss. As a species, our bodies are programmed to retain calories and store them away in our fat for long winters or famine: conditions that rarely exist today. In fact, our bodies actually become more efficient at storing away calories when we diet. The reason being is that it presumes a decrease in our caloric intake is the result of environmental conditions leading to decreases in food sources. This is why dieting is such an uphill battle: not only are we fighting our own poor eating habits, but our own human physiology. HCG flips this upside down allowing us to sustain ourselves on our own stored fat.

Why such a low calorie diet?

The calorie restrictions and elimination of carbs are what results in your weight loss. The HCG merely targets and unlocks your abnormal fat reserves that are stored in our problem areas so we maintain muscle mass and healthy fat stores. See below.

How is the HCG protocol different from any other diet out there?

Dr. Simeons, the physician who developed the *HCG Weight Loss Protocol*, said in his manuscript, ***Pounds and Inches;*** *A New Approach to Obesity*, "When an obese patient tries to reduce by starving himself, he will first lose his normal fat reserves. When these are exhausted he begins to burn up structural fat, and only as a last resort will the body yield its abnormal reserves, though by that time the patient usually feels so weak and hungry that the diet is abandoned. It is just for this reason that obese patients complain that when they diet they lose the wrong fat. They feel famished and tired and their face becomes drawn and haggard, but their belly, hips, thighs and upper arms show little improvement. The fat they have come to detest stays on and the fat they need to cover their bones gets less and less. Their skin wrinkles and they look old and miserable. And that is one of the most frustrating and depressing experiences a human being can have."

To paraphrase Dr. Simeons, HCG allows you to tap into your body's abnormal fat deposits (shoulders, upper arms, hips, thighs, and buttocks). In obese patients, these deposits are not usually accessible to the body until the person has gone through both his normal fat and structural fat as described above. This is the reason why no matter how much some people exercise and starve him/her; they are still incapable of shedding their unwanted weight. The HCG, coupled with the low calorie diet, as outlined in HCG 2.0, allows these abnormal fat deposits to be used by the dieter as a calorie source thus sustaining themselves on their own stored fat while maintaining muscle mass.

What will I eat on this protocol?

It's recommended that you eat healthy whole food diet of primarily lean protein. Refer to you chart listing your protein items ranked from best to adequate using the calculation below. The higher the P/CF a protein sources has the more you'll be able to eat of that particular protein. For example, you could have 3.5 oz of chicken breast or 7 oz of Tilapia. You have a lot more options on this diet than you do with the traditional HCG Diet.

How does this program compare to others?

The chart below is a time vs. cost comparison in losing 20lbs. Also keep in mind that HCG dieters tend to lose several inches from problem areas: generally about 1 to 1.5 inches per pound. I had a women recently that was disappointed she only lost 19 pounds, but after measuring she lost of total of 39 inches. That's over 3 feet! This will make a tremendous difference in the way your clothes fit. Shopping makes a perfect reward for a job well done.

Weight Loss Program	Average amount of time needed to lose 20 lbs.	Cost
Weight Watchers	12 Weeks	$120
Medifast 5-1 Plan	6 Weeks	$650
Nutri System	12 Weeks	$900
Jenny Craig	12 Weeks	$1,250
Traditional HCG Diet	5 Weeks	$100 Non-Prescription $400 Prescription
HCG 2.0	5 Weeks	$100 Non-Prescription $400 Prescription

About the Author

Dr. Zach LaBoube, Chiropractor and Fellow of the American Society of Acupuncture, is completing a Master's of Science in Nutrition and Human Performance from Logan University. He founded InsideOut Wellness and Weight Loss with the belief that true health radiates, fundamentally, from the inside out. You can visit his blog at www.insideoutwellness.net.

Additional HCG 2.0 Diet Tools Available at...

www.InsideOutWellness.net
www.Facebook.com/hcg2.0

Enter promo code **AMAZON** to have the cost of your book deducted from your HCG 2.0 purchase.

Bibliography

de Aquino , L., Pereira, S., de Souza , S. J., Sobrinho , C., & Ramalho , A. (2012). Bariatric surgery: impact on body composition after roux-en-y gastric bypass.*Pub.Med.gov*, Retrieved from http://www.ncbi.nlm.nih.gov/pubmed/21881836

Farias, M., Cuevas, A., & Rodriguez, F. (2011). Set point theory and obesity. *PubMed.gov*, Retrieved from www.ncbi.nlm.nih.gov/m/pubmed/21117971/

Freedhoff, Y. (2007, June 14). [Web log message]. Retrieved from http://www.weightymatters.ca/2007/06/set-point-theory.html

Moore, J. (2007, January 7). *I knew it! low-carb inuit diet protects against heart disease, cancer, study finds*. Retrieved from http://livinlavidalowcarb.com/blog/i-knew-it-low-carb-inuit-diet-protects-against-heart-disease-cancer-study-finds/1467

Oz, D. M. (2011, June 27). Imagine losing a pound a day but never feeling hungry. *For women First*

Prinster, L. (2007). *Hcg weight loss cure guide*. (5th ed.). USA: Everything Matters Publishing.

Simeons, A. T. W. (1954). *Pounds and inches: A new approach to obesity*. Jump Start Publishing.

University of Wisconsin (n.d.). *Hypothalamus*. Retrieved from http://www.neuroanatomy.wisc.edu/coursebook/neuro2(2).pdf

Zaleson, K., Franklin, B., Lillystone, M., Shamon, T., Krause, K., Chengelis, D., Mucci, S., & Shaheen, K. (2010). Differential loss of fat and lean mass in the morbidly obese after bariatric surgery.*Pub.Med.gov*, Retrieved from http://www.ncbi.nlm.nih.gov/pubmed/19929598

Notes

9 781490 964164